Individualism and Families

Almost all women and men claim that gender equality within their relationships is the ideal. In practice, however, equality is not predominant within many couples and families. This book develops current debates about individualisation within families – particularly how partners understand and resolve tensions between the need for togetherness and personal autonomy, and how partners view and work with increasing gender equality.

Individualism and Families is based on an in depth Swedish study from two of the foremost European experts on the sociology of the family. The study looks particularly at partnering, parenting, intimacy, commitments, attitudes to finances and gender divisions of labour.

This book will be invaluable reading for academics and students in sociology, family studies, gender studies and other applied social sciences.

Ulla Björnberg is Professor of Sociology at the University of Göteborg, Sweden and is well known internationally as an expert in the comparative sociology of family life and family policy.

Anna-Karin Kollind is Lecturer and Researcher in Family Sociology, in the Department of Sociology, University of Göteborg. She has conducted research on stepfamilies, on the social history of family counselling in Sweden and, with Ulla Björnberg, on dual-earner couples.

Individualism and Families

Equality, autonomy and togetherness

Ulla Björnberg and Anna-Karin Kollind

Routledge
Taylor & Francis Group

LONDON AND NEW YORK

First published in 2005 by Routledge
2 Park Square, Milton Park, Abingdon, Oxon OX14 4RN

Simultaneously published in the USA and Canada
by Routledge
711 Third Avenue, New York, NY 10017

Routledge is an imprint of the Taylor & Francis Group, an informa business

© 2005 Ulla Björnberg and Anna-Karin Kollind

Typeset in 10 point Sabon MT by J&L Composition, Filey,
North Yorkshire

British Library Cataloguing in Publication Data
A catalogue record for this book is available from the British
Library

Library of Congress Cataloging in Publication Data
A catalogue record for this book has been requested

ISBN 0-415-34363-1 (hbk)
ISBN 0-415-34364-X (pbk)

Contents

Preface

The work associated with writing this book has been made possible through financial support from the Swedish Council for Working Life and Social Research. The translation, by Åsa Björnberg, has been financed by a grant from The Foundation Wilhelm and Martina Lundgren Science Fund. We are very grateful for this support. We would also like to send a heartfelt thank you to the women and men who participated in the study, who let us share their experiences upon which this book is created. It is our hope that these experiences and our analyses will inspire readers to think about how equality, autonomy and togetherness are managed in everyday life. In the public discourse, equality is usually portrayed in terms of equal sharing. Our analyses show that equality in couple relationships can be perceived in a multitude of ways. Creating equality in everyday life entails much more than sharing equally. With this book, it is our desire to increase the understanding of how gender differences are perpetuated – and of how they are transgressed.

This project has been collaborative, and all the chapters have been processed by both authors. Anna-Karin Kollind has been chiefly responsible for Chapters 2, 3, 5 and 6, and Ulla Björnberg for Chapters 4, 7, 8 and 9.

Chapter 1

Introduction

What does equality in couple relationships mean? Almost all women and men claim that a gender equality ideal is a matter of course. Despite this, gender equality is not predominant in many couple relationships. There are many reasons for this difference in both thought and action, and we want to emphasise this problem. The view of individuals as separate and independent, with special interests and needs, is integrated in the equality ideal. In the notion of the family, however, togetherness is viewed as basic, and the individuals are seen as giving priority to what best serves the family. Families governed by equality thus necessitate both independence and subordination in relation to togetherness. Being able to unify these two is the great challenge for couples nowadays.

This book describes how women and men manage issues of togetherness and equality in their family relations. We will demonstrate conflicts met by women and men in their everyday life while trying to unify the ideals of equality and togetherness. The issue of equality touches a deeper level that concerns the actual meaning of family for individuals in modern society. The concept of 'family' is multifaceted, and subject to many interpretations. It can include many types of relationships and bonds. When talking about the family, we can refer to biological kinship in the broader sense. We may also refer to people who we have added to 'our family', even if there are no biological connections. Certain family relationships seem to prevail, in the sense that they are regarded as lifelong, regardless of the quality of the relationship. These are true of children, parents and siblings. Elderly parents do not cease referring to their children as children even when these children have become grey haired and are retired. From the life perspective of the individual, family ties are subject to change in terms of content and significance. Yet, we often associate the word 'family' with one man, one woman and their children all belonging together, that is, the nuclear family. In our study, this is the type of family in focus, women and men who live together and have school-age children of their own. This focus is not because we think that this family type is representative of the only 'genuine' family. It is a result of our interest in investigating how cohesion is created and maintained in relationships where couples have lived together for a relatively large number of years.

Every time a couple is formed, ties are created irrespectively of whether the couple is hetero- or homosexual. These ties are based on ideas of togetherness and cohesion, yet, the more detailed implications of these ideas are not necessarily very clear to the involved parties. The partners may also have different ideas on these issues. Granted, there are general ideas and norms regarding what family cohesion means in each society, but they are neither compulsory nor particularly straightforward in this society. Every couple is entitled to formulate their own special rules for their 'unity', guided by their own norms, experiences and ideals. 'Own' rules are created by each couple. In practice, this means that obligations and rights towards each other are the result of compromise. In this study, we want to show different ways in which the circumstances for togetherness are created.

Since the mid-1980s, researchers have claimed that the character of family ties in modern society have become increasingly temporary. For example, claims have been made that the family as an institution has been converted from a moral-social contract to a more personal project (Théry 1993). This implies more open agreements made by the parties, that later may become subject to negotiation (Godbout 1992; Giddens 1992). According to these researchers, the family thus becomes a social institution, which is decreasingly based on moral concepts regarding obligations and rights related to a certain position. This supposition claims that present-day couples can create more varied forms of togetherness compared to what was previously possible. Therefore, patterns for duties and obligations are neither given nor predictable.

For many people, it is no longer obvious that the woman takes care of the home and the household, while the man is responsible for the breadwinning. It is also no longer self-evident that small children are women's domain of responsibility, and that the role of men becomes engaged only when the children are older. Yet, even if such gender-specific obligations are no longer taken for granted, many studies point to differences of ideals and practices. Women often carry the chief responsibility for the home, household and children. Men work full time and women cut down on their time in wage labour. In the practical formulation of the daily intercourse, routines and division of responsibility and labour, the gender divide is still determined, even in relatively young families. At the same time, changes are taking place in the relationship between the genders, often at a slow pace and in ways that are hard to grasp. There are still conflicts in the home about washing the dishes, doing the cleaning, driving the children around and staying at home with the children when they are ill.

The cohabiting partners cannot avoid the creation of rules for the coexistence in the home. How are they going to deal with the ongoing chores in a shared household? And how should they deal with e.g. home improvement – is that responsibility up to one or both parties? Other central issues concern the relationship to children (if there are any), as well as keeping contact with friends and relatives. How should they manage parental leave, childcare, rules concerning what the children may or may not have? Should both parties carry this responsibility, or should the responsibility and the decisions be shared? What guidelines should apply? All of the above relates to care for objects, persons and relationships. The solutions developed by couples include issues of allocation, in other words who spends time and effort on specific things. Other important issues of allocation include money and time. What does a reasonable distribution of time at work and at leisure look like? What is perceived as fair and unfair?

The cohesion in a couple relationship is based on love and a desire to be together. Yet daily affairs concerning work, time and money are also important components in this togetherness. Through decisions, compromise and habitual actions, explicit and implicit rules take shape around obligations and rights. In these processes, relationships of dominance are created, often at the unconscious level. Our provisional label for this is *negotiations*. The significance of this will be discussed in later chapters of this book.

In the allocation of love, money, time, work and influence, two themes inevitably emerge. One of the themes concerns independence or autonomy, the space accessible to each party in terms of his/her own needs and wishes. The partner who is continually being questioned about what he/she is going to do or is thinking about may perceive him/herself as controlled, and that there is a lack of personal autonomy in the relationship. The individual in a couple who asks him/herself 'What about me, is there no space for my needs?' is struggling with the imbalance between togetherness and autonomy. A partial aim of this study is to shed light on how couples reason around the needs of autonomy and togetherness that are accentuated in each couple relationship, and how they handle the tensions that surface.

The second theme is about gender equality, which since the mid-1970s has become an ideal in society. It has become a political goal as well as a central theme of discourse in a multitude of societal contexts. Ideals of equality have become integrated in practical politics and have influenced legislation and education. The ideals have also given rise to action plans in the workplace etc. Our position is that no couple can avoid relating to these ideals. You can reject or accept them, and try to translate them into practice. We claim that the meaning attributed to the ideal of gender equality is far from transparent in terms of how it is perceived and how it is converted into practice in actual situations in couple relationships.

The themes that we regard to be important in this context is how couples with children living together handle issues of togetherness and independence, and how they relate to gender equality as an ideal and as a practice.

The study and its participants

This study is based on interviews with twenty-two parent couples, all of whom are in paid work. The interviews were carried out in 1997 as a follow-up of a larger study sample of 670 families with children. This larger study was carried out in 1992, with the purpose of creating an overview of how parents in differ-ent socio-economic situations viewed their possibilities of combining paid work with family life, and which family policies they regarded as particularly urgent.[1] The parents' view of the children, conflicts regarding children and money as well as division of household labour were also studied.[2] The parents inter-viewed in 1992 were asked if they were willing to be interviewed in more depth. Slightly more than 90 per cent said yes. Five years later, we made a new selec-tion on the basis of these replies. The new sample was not random but selective, particularly with reference to profession, but also restricted to the city of Gothenburg.

The follow-up study presented in this book covers three main areas. First, we focus on allocation of work in the household, as well as paid and unpaid work. Household labour includes caring for children. Second, we examine the alloca-tion of money between the partners,[3] room for shared and private consumption and saving, as well as decisions regarding household purchases. Third, we discuss conflict management and issues of influence.

A question guide was used in the interviews. The guide was developed by both researchers, but the interviews were carried out individually. In the devel-opment of the questionnaire, we strived to obtain a shared understanding of the purpose with each question, so that the questions would lead to similar associations in the respondents. Pilot test-interviews led to amendments of the question guide, which subsequently remained intact. Our approach was to adopt a conversational tone in the interviews.

We also used a vignette technique in the interviews. This consisted of printed cards describing moral problems in everyday situations that couples may face. The vignette was read aloud to the participants, who were asked to describe how she or he thought the problem ought to be solved and give arguments why. The next step for the participant was to say whether the situation was similar to anything they had experienced. The participants often provided spontaneous examples taken from their own lives, and described how the problems were solved. In the interviews, we aimed to extract moral arguments for the choice of solution to such issues. The purpose was to study how arguments about mutuality (reciprocity) gain expression.

Men and women were interviewed separately, usually in their home. A few interviews were carried out in our offices at the university. The interviews lasted anything between one and three hours, with a typical duration of two hours. Tape recorders were used in the interviews, and the recordings were transcribed word for word. The interviews were analysed from different thematic angles, categorisation and coding created stepwise from broad to narrow categories. During the coding, quotes that provide illuminating thematic examples were extracted and used as illustrations and evidence. Thematic analyses were achieved by repeated thematic reading of the transcripts and noting down results and interpretations. This work was carried out in parallel, and results and interpretations were discussed in detail. The work was time-consuming, but provided reliability, since both researchers worked through all interview transcripts separately. In our view, this method has ensured reliability in terms of interpretation and analysis of the material.

The interviewed couples had lived together for approximately ten years. In view of the divorce statistics, they can be regarded as being successful couples. According to Swedish statistics, 23 per cent of married couples divorce after ten years of living together, and after fifteen years, the percentage of divorce is 30. The risk of separation is even higher for unmarried couples who live together (Statstics Sweden, 1995).

Our primary interest in the study focuses on the strategies employed by women and men in managing issues of division of labour, money and influence. Conflicts are live elements in the everyday lives of couples, although most try to avoid open confrontation.

Income, work and social background are important factors to consider when studying equality in couple relationships. The party with a higher income may have a greater influence on division of labour in the home or in terms of jointly shared and separate consumption. Circumstances of upbringing may also have an effect on the resources contributed to the household. Similarly, professional status can influence negotiations between the spouses concerning allocation of time and work. The person with higher professional status could claim that the work demands being present in different ways, such as commitments with colleagues after work, travelling or being flexible.

The sample of families consisted of established couples whose children were above toddler age. Sixteen of the couples had two children in the household, four had one child and two had three children. The majority of children were between the ages of 8 and 10 years old. The parents represented both the middle and working classes. Service professions were predominant, but other professions were also included in the sample. All parents were in paid work, but almost half of the women worked part time in various forms. The women were predominantly employed by the public sector, the men in the private sector. Five of the women had compulsory education only (nine years); the rest had college or university education. More than half of the men had college or university education, the rest had some kind of professional education.[4]

Book outline

The three chapters following this introduction present the theoretical perspectives that have guided the analyses of our most important themes – division of labour, allocation of money and conflict management.

Chapter 2 presents the theoretical viewpoints used to analyse gender equality. Furthermore, different definitions of gender equality based on various research approaches are discussed.

Chapter 3 focuses on the relationship between autonomy and togetherness, the binding factor of the entire subsequent interview analysis. Theories of social togetherness and various aspects on how forms of togetherness are created and maintained are also included in this chapter. We differentiate between various forms of togetherness and the superior logics that guide them. In conjunction, we also discuss rights and obligations in various types of togetherness.

Chapter 4 is about perceptions of ethics and morals, and how these form the binding factor in the creation of both togetherness and equality. The tensions between independence and togetherness in the management of conflicting interests are also discussed here. We also touch upon different models of conflict resolution in this chapter.

The results of the interviews are described in Chapters 5 and 6, where we present different aspects of division of labour. The tensions between the ideal and actual divisions of labour that take place in practice are highlighted in Chapter 5, while Chapter 6 sheds light on equality ideals, and how these are reflected in various ways of speaking of and practising equality. Furthermore, different principles for accomplishing equality in division of labour are scrutinised. Chapter 6 ends with a description of three strategies of division of labour.

Chapter 7 shows how the couples allocate money and property, and the reasoning about consumption and saving. This chapter also describes the relationship between the ideal and the actual. It gives an account of different patterns of managing individual and jointly shared needs in the household economy. In addition, the decision-making processes behind purchasing and saving are illuminated.

Chapter 8 describes how couples manage oppositions and create boundaries, for example regarding the children and demands on time to oneself. We differentiate between styles of managing conflicts, and discuss what significance these may have in the creation of togetherness and equality.

Chapter 9 consists of a summary of the results and an analysis of the main themes – the relationship between equality, autonomy and togetherness.

Chapter 2

Gender equality in families

Family and equality

A core theme in this study is the equality of family life. What values are associated with equality, and how are they converted into practice? What does equality mean to people in their everyday lives? Is equality considered to be important in family life? How are discrepancies between ideal and reality handled? These questions derive from our interest in understanding not only what factors contribute to the reproduction of gender-determined boundaries, but also how they are transcended.

Equality as a political vision

The issue of equality has been an integrated part of both national and international politics since the 1970s. During this decade, the first international women's conferences were held, and in 1979, the United Nations issued a convention against all forms of discrimination of women. In Sweden, a Delegation for Equality between Men and Women was formed in 1972. In 1974 the Instrument of Government stipulated that 'the public will assure equal rights of men and women' and that no individual should be 'disadvantaged on the basis of sex' (§1:2, §2:16 in Petrén and Ragnemalm, 1980). By 1979, Sweden had its first law of equality. Since the 1970s, the issue has also become more formal in its character, inasmuch as a cabinet minister was appointed with special responsibility for equality politics. In due course, this ministerial post was also given a separate unit within the department. There are now equality committees on several levels in society (see e.g. Fürst 2000).

There is substantial political unity regarding equality as an ideal, although the practical politics may vary significantly. Through legislation and other political action, politicians have wanted to promote equality in working life and in education. One goal has been *equal gender distribution* in all sectors of society. The criterion was established to be between 40 and 60 per cent for women and men respectively. One way of reaching this goal has been through applying quotas. Quotas for males have been assigned to female-dominated educations and vice versa. Other means to counter skewness in the gender distribution have consisted of the requirement for equality plans laid out by workplaces and schools. Equality ideals have also affected family policies to a certain extent. When individual taxation was introduced in 1971, it was motivated by the fact that joint taxation provided worse conditions for married women in terms of paid labour compared to those of men and unmarried women. When the maternity benefit was renamed 'parental insurance', it was a symbolic statement saying that the care for small children is not exclusively a female preoccupation, but something that should concern both parents. Women's and men's right to share the parental leave was another step in that direction. The so-called 'daddy months', i.e. two months' leave within the framework of parental leave that are exclusively retained for the father, is another example of how the equality ideal has been converted into political practice.

The goal of equality politics is to clear out factors that contribute to gender segregation and gender-based discrimination. The view is that it is vital that women have the same opportunities as men to govern and control their life conditions. The aim is that both men and women should have equal opportunities, that choices should be governed by individual preferences and not by unequal conditions. Equal opportunities can be made real through such things as equal rights to education, career, equal salaries for equal work and shared responsibility for the home and children.

The positive esteem of equality politics in the public discourse does not naturally lead to a general acceptance of the equality ideals. Gender-based salary discrimination, sexual harassment and gender-stereotypical verbal abuse, rape and wife beating, male dominance in most leading positions are only a few examples testifying that the ideal is anchored in fragile grounds to a higher extent than the official ideology purports.

Several studies of families that are now considered as 'classics' deal with issues related to processes of change towards a greater equality between spouses, sometimes referred to as the process of democratisation in the intimate sphere. When Burgess and Locke in the 1940s claimed that the family was changing from being an institution to becoming a companionship, they were referring to the move towards a greater equality (Burgess and Locke 1945). This was also the case for Young and Willmotts' (1973) study about changes towards a more symmetrical family, as well as the development of the dual-earner family (Rapoport and Rapoport 1976). Women's paid labour was thought to clear the way for a greater equality in the family.

Swedish family policy in brief

In the 1970s some important reforms were introduced in Sweden in order to promote equal opportunities for women. With these reforms an 'adult worker family model' was institutionalised in society.[1] These reforms were integrated into a more encompassing model of the Swedish welfare state after the Second World War which has been characterised as a universalistic model with individual and gender neutral social rights and with an extended responsibility of the public for social care and social services.[2] Financial independence between men and women in the family is a cornerstone in the adult worker family model. Social insurances such as unemployment benefits and sickness benefits are related to the income of the insured person. Pensions are based on the individual incomes during the life course. Taxes are paid by the individual, unrelated to the income of his or her partner. Lone mothers are treated as breadwinners in their own right. They are expected to be in paid work and they are supported through affordable childcare provided to all children. Children of divorced or separated parents can receive a maintenance allowance (Swedish Code of Statutes, 1996: 1031) that is advanced by the state in the amount of 128 € a month. The age limit is set at the age of 18 or 20 if the child is still in school. A parent who is ordered to pay maintenance allowance has to repay to the state according to economic ability, some of the 128 € or all of it, depending on income. Child allowance is granted to all children below 16 years old, regardless of the incomes of the parents. In 2004 the child allowance was 104 € a month. It is expected to cover one-third of the direct costs of having a pre-school child, and one-fifth of the cost of a teenager (Ministry of Health and Social Affairs 2001; (Ds 2001: 57). Child allowance is given to all children up until age 16, and then student aid is paid at the same amount for those who continue in education (which most children currently do) up until age 20, but then only during nine months a year (the school year).[3]

A means-tested housing allowance is also available to families with children in Sweden. It is calculated on the basis of the housing cost and the number of children in the household, and then calculated against the estimated income during the coming year.

Both women and men as parents have a right to parental leave with income replacement. The leave period for either parent is 480 days; 390 days are covered by income replacement of 80 per cent up to an income level of roughly 70 € a day and 90 days with a flat rate amount of about 17 € a day. Parental leave is a right, which is individual. However, most available days (except for two months) can be transferred to one parent: it is not regarded as an individualised right, but as a family right. Mothers use about 85 per cent of the available days.

The rules of parental leave allow for flexibility in how leave is used since parents can share days. Under the same legislation parents are entitled to 60 days leave per child (below 12 years) per year if the child or the childminder is sick. Additionally, fathers are entitled to ten days' paternity leave after birth under the same income replacement rate as parental leave.

Public childcare has been an important part of the reform programme, but provision of public childcare became mandatory for municipalities only in 1995. In 2001 71 per cent of pre-school children and 35 per cent of school children below 12 years were enrolled in day-care institutions. Childcare provided through the private market accounts for only a minor share – 12 per cent in 1999 (but still an increase from 4 per cent in 1990) (Statistics Sweden 2003).

Altogether, in terms of gender aspects of social citizenship, the Swedish system can be categorised as a defamilised system defined as the degree to which women have the capacity to form independent households and that the public sector provide services for care of dependent family members to enable women to engage in paid work (Daly 2000; Lister 2003). At a formal level, women are granted autonomy in the sense that they enjoy a high degree of freedom in relation to family for income and services. Income maintenance is provided through different support systems (social insurances) that primarily are based on individual entitlements.

Slow processes of change

In an international perspective, the Swedish institutional regulations of the 'adult worker family' in terms of individual taxation, parental leave, public provision of care of dependent children, elderly and disabled family members, provide conditions for equal gender relations. In international comparisons of gender equality on indicators of paid work and political participation, Sweden and other countries with similar institutional arrangements display relatively higher degree of gender equality compared with countries with other models (Korpi 2000). Studies that have been comparing Swedish patterns of sharing domestic work and care with those in other countries have pointed at relatively more gender equality in the home than are found between countries (Crompton 1999; Anxo 2003; Sundström 2003; Takahashi 2003). In these studies it has been argued that Swedish laws and welfare institutions have brought egalitarian gender practices and attitudes and encouraged women to claim equal division of labour in the household. However, despite these institutionalised rights, gender inequality in the labour market and in domestic chores and childcare are persistent and changing only at a slow pace at least when looked upon in a national frame of reference.

Repeated investigations and statistics have shown, however, that women live in worse economic and social conditions than men. Their incomes are lower, they perform more unpaid labour, they often have subordinate positions in the workplace and their time is to a larger extent constrained by set structures. Women have the greatest responsibility for children and the family, for the planning and coordination of the children's schedule with those of their partners and themselves. Children and family responsibilities mean that a large proportion of adult women do not work full time, which in turn leads to more limited finances and, in the long term, a more limited pension. The man is still regarded as the main breadwinner of the family, and he has a greater possibility of deciding the conditions for his efforts in the home (see for example Haavind 1987; Andersson 1993; Holmberg 1993; Bäck-Wiklund and Bergsten 1997; Björnberg 1997; Magnusson 1998; Plantin 2001).

A study on time use of labour in households with children showed the following results in 1991: in households with older school children, the women performed on average twenty-one hours per week in household work, whereas the men performed just over five hours. The difference was thus more than fifteen hours. The time spent on paid labour was approximately forty hours for the men and thirty-four hours for the women, a difference of six hours. This means that the average total number of working hours was fifty-five for women and forty-five for men. These figures are aggregated, and thus provide only a rough overall estimate. However, the main message is clear: women's total time spent working is greater than that of men, while their incomes are lower, and these differences increase with the age of the children. When comparing the situation in 1991 with that of 1974, we see that women aged about 35 spend dramatically less time performing household labour, from forty to twenty hours per week. The men have increased their time somewhat – from three to approximately five. In this comparison, no differences are made between households with or without children; it accounts only for the working time of women and men who are aged 35 (Hörnqvist 1997).

On the whole, it can be said that women's working hours, wage development and career opportunities are affected negatively by having children and a family, whereas for men, these factors are affected in a very minor way.

Formally, policies provide equal opportunities for men and women, but for different reasons, a rather traditional pattern remains in family life. How we perceive this change is, however, dependent on how we study these issues and where the focus lies. Even though the pattern shows that women's responsibility for the household is dominant, studies also show significant differences in equality among couples. One example of this is Ahrne and Roman's (1997) study, where approximately 13 per cent of the couples were considered as equal, and almost 25 per cent were considered to be partially equal (semi-equal). The criterion for equality was that the couples shared equally chores such as cooking, washing and cleaning, or that the man did 'more in one or more of these chores' and the woman more of something else (Ahrne and Roman 1997: 28). Several studies have shown that men's relationship with the family is transformed through fatherhood and that the number of fathers who take paternal leave is increasing (Plantin 2001; Chronholm 2002). It seems as though changes are taking place. Femininity and masculinity no longer determine tasks to the same extent, and the space for negotiation is greater.

Norms concerning good motherhood, however, still determine the priorities that men and women make during the years when the child is in the home. These priorities are reinforced by the labour market. It is expected that men are work oriented and career driven, whereas women are expected to be family oriented. Women are thus given opportunities of flexible working hours and part-time work. Some of the adaptations that occur in people's relationships and the surrounding systems oppose the changes intended by political reform (Magnusson 1998; Plantin 2001; Björnberg 2002).

In every society, norms, behaviours and attitudes are constructed on gender, with socially significant consequences – such as a gendered labour market, salary levels and working conditions that are determined by gender, to mention a few. A differentiation takes place that outlines the separation between the genders. A gender order not only places a difference between the male and the female, but also creates a rank order between what is better and worse, higher and lower. The inherent hierarchy of the gender order creates constraining circumstances for social relations, and it is within these 'constraints' that 'gender' is created.[4]

'Doing gender' means choosing actions that confirm one's notions of what is 'correct' from a gender perspective (Fenstermacher et al. 1991). Normative conceptions of how gender works in everyday life act as guidelines. They are thus not given, but negotiable and changeable. Transcending normative gender expectations implicates a challenge of the gender power. The person who goes against the gender norms can expect reactions from the surrounding environment. Whether you go against these norms or not, the individual becomes accountable to him or herself for the choices made. This perspective accentuates the fact that people construct gender first and foremost through their actions.

Gender equality – in which families?

The dominant picture provided by the research presented so far is one of slow, structural and institutional change, as well as slow changes in thought processes and behaviour patterns. Below we will present a number of studies, Swedish and international, that focus directly on aspects of equality in family life. We will also discuss how these studies have interpreted and defined equality, since this definition is by no means universal. Our chief interest in this section is thus equality as a normative concept.

Division of labour in the household is one of the most common areas in family oriented equality research. The common denominator of these studies is the attempt to provide an overview of how time and work is allocated between men and women who live together. Our purpose is to extract the basis of the assumptions made about equality in these studies. All these studies focus on similarities and differences in the amount of time and work men and women spend in household labour. Ahrne and Roman's (1997) study mentioned above is an example of this. The family typology developed in this study – equal, semi-equal, conventional and patriarchal – was based on the spouses' way of sharing chores like washing, cleaning and cooking. Couples who spent equal amounts of time doing these chores were considered to be equal. Equality was thus measured in terms of sameness in work and time. There is a certain amount of agreement between this definition of equality in couple relationships and legislated equality. Both take account of equal conditions and possibilities for women and men. Efforts made towards having as many men and women in different lines of education, professions and decision-making bodies reflect a distributive equality. Our purpose is not to criticise politics or this particular view of equality. Instead, our purpose is to discuss how gender equality in family life can be defined.

There are some studies of equality in couple relationships that are based on different definitions. One example is a study by Schwartz (1994), who used several criteria when judging equality. In addition to amounts of time spent on household work, power and influence were also important criteria. A balanced influence on important issues regarding the family's situation was part of the definition of an equal marriage. Both parties should have equal control over the family's economic resources, have the same economic independence, and the work performed by each party should be regarded as having equal value. In Schwartz's (1994) study, allocation of time was not a sufficient criterion of equality, but allocation of control or influence was also viewed as significant. A similar perspective can be found in Holmberg's (1993) study of young, childless couples, although it contains no explicit definition of equality. Holmberg's interest was to show that couples who thought themselves to be equal, and were also regarded as equal by others, still remained directed by principles of superiority and subordination of the genders. The criterion for equality in this perspective is the absence of gender-determined mechanisms of superiority and subordination (Holmberg 1993). A similar approach has been used by Roman (1999).

In another American study of equality, Risman and Johnson-Sumerford (1998) asked married couples if they considered their division of labour, money, time and care for the children to be fair and equal. In addition to criteria such as equality in terms of actual allocation of time, labour and money, the researchers took into account the couples' own perceptions of whether they were living in an equal relationship. This aspect was even more central in work performed by Knudson-Martin and Mahoney (1998). They were interested in how couples construct equality and brought attention to the way in which cohabiting men and women spoke about issues of equality. By listening to cohabiting couples' conversations, the researchers attempted to read into and analyse the construction of an equal relationship. They discerned three signs used by couples in the conversations that demonstrated equality. The signs mentioned were mutual adaptation, mutual attention and a shared experience of well-being.

All in all, these studies show that equality in couple relationships can be defined in different ways, and a definition can include one or more dimensions. It may focus on aspects of sameness, the degree of sameness in allocation of time and labour, burdens and privileges. It may emphasise the presence or absence of power, influence or control. It can also take into account aspects of mutuality between the parties and include their own experiences of living in an equal relationship.

Definition of equality thus constitutes a pivotal question in these kinds of studies. In the examples mentioned above, it is usually the researchers who create the definition that the study is based upon or that the results are evaluated according to. The exception is that of Knudson-Martin and Mohoney (1998), whose basic perspective is how couples themselves construct the definition of equality.

A Swedish study with a similar perspective was carried out by the ethnologist Lena Martinsson (1997). She presents ten couples and their ways of reasoning and thinking about equality. Martinsson's interest is not whether the participants are equal or not, nor is she interested in how equality should or could be defined. She claims that norms of equality are coercive, to the extent that most people in society are unable to avoid relating to gender issues. Constant talks about gender, femininity and masculinity shape human understanding of the self and thus also of gender. The equality discourse that goes on in all kinds of contexts is not fixed, unambiguous, complete or possible to restrict. The discourse affects people's perceptions of gender. Martinsson sheds light on the actual narrative about equality, what people do with it and what it does to them (Martinsson 1997: 84).

According to Martinsson (1997), we are a long way from knowing exactly how norms of equality will be understood, what meaning will be attached to it and how it is put into practice in the lives of human beings. There were women in the couples interviewed by her whose thoughts on equality and demands on independence had made them choose to stay at home with the children instead of working for some 'bloke'. They refused to subordinate themselves to male gender hierarchies in the workplace. These women claimed to have chosen home-making in order to safeguard their freedom and independence. In other words, they had caught on to certain parts of the equality discourse, given them meaningful attributes and had also reached an understanding of themselves, their motives and their actions through the discourse (Martinsson 1997: 109–110). According to Martinsson, it is difficult to predetermine what implications discourses of equality ideals might have and how women and men choose to apply them in their situations in life.

Martinsson never attempts to provide a general definition of equality. In this respect, her work is different from that of the others, who all make the assumption that it is possible and meaningful to ascertain criteria for what is meant by equality. Based on these studies, two perspectives can be discerned. From one perspective, the researcher defines the concept of equality, often according to officially accepted principles. In the other perspective, the participants themselves define equality by expressing their thoughts. In our view, the first perspective is 'external'. Criteria of equality are determined by researchers (or general discourses, laws or ordinances). People's descriptions of how they behave and think are in this case judged according to predetermined criteria. We name the other perspective 'internal'. In this case, the participants' judgement of what equality means to them determines the understanding.

Martinsson's (1997) and Knudson-Martin and Mahoney's (1998) studies are clear cases of the 'internal' perspective. To a certain extent, this is also the case for Risman and Johnson-Sumerford (1998), since they consider it important to take into account how the involved parties reflect on their own situation. The remaining studies, on the other hand, apply more of an 'external' perspective.

In this study, we are interested to find out how the interviewees perceive equality. What does equality imply for them? We are also interested in how equality is valued as a norm. Is equality positive? Is it something of importance, or does it not concern them very much? We also want to understand the interviewees' representations of equality in the family. In this sense, we have utilised an internal perspective. It is not relevant for us to assess equality in the relationships according to predetermined principles. Rather, it is relevant to find out what equality represent in their lives.

Arlie Hochschild's (1989) book *The Second Shift* provides an example of a methodology that includes both the internal and the external perspectives. She uses case descriptions to shed light on different strategies of managing equality issues. One of the cases concerns a woman who had had plenty of previous conflicts with her husband concerning division of labour in the home. Eventually, they resolved the conflict and reached a pact of mutual understanding. The conflict resolution entailed that the woman was responsible for all 'upstairs' work, and the man was responsible for all work 'downstairs'. That which is implicit or non-verbal from the external perspective was the notion that 'upstairs' referred to all floors above the cellar (the kitchen, living room, bedroom and bathroom), whereas 'downstairs' referred only to the cellar, which the husband used as a hobby room. From an external perspective, this is an unequal division of domestic work. However, from the internal perspective, she explains how this model maintained the couple's image of themselves as being 'equal'.

Hochschild's (1989) study is an example of research that aims to highlight the slowness of changes in family patterns towards equality. She highlights the sometimes unconscious strategies used by couples to avoid seeing obvious discrepancies between their ideals of equality and the actual practice of everyday life. In order to understand how couples such as the above can uphold such collusions, it is necessary for Hochschild to use the internal perspective. She must understand the man's and the woman's reasoning. At the same time, it is also necessary to use the external perspective, i.e. distance oneself from the couple's perspective and judge their equality based on other criteria.

In our own study, we have similarly made an attempt to apply and combine the two perspectives, internal and external. The latter implies that we have avoided classifying the interviewed couples based on a definition of equality of our own choice. Instead, the interviewees' judgement of themselves as equal couples provides the basis for classification. Our interest here has been to find out how they think about equality, and what they include in the concept. However, the analyses have sometimes pointed to great discrepancies between how equal the individuals consider themselves to be and their descriptions of their everyday lives. When such evaluations are made, they apply a definition of equality. Criteria that we regard as important for the creation of equality are then used. These criteria are a presence of mutuality in the division of resources and work, space for individual power and a possibility to make choices without being forced. Furthermore, it is important that there is a balance of power and influence in the household. We think that equality should be viewed as a process, a way of relating to one another, rather than a result. In the following chapters, we will define these conditions and concepts in more detail.

At this point, it should be absolutely clear that the issue of equality is one of our themes. Other themes of equal importance are togetherness and individual autonomy, and their implications in everyday life. Togetherness, autonomy and equality are not independent of each other, but connected in various patterns. This has consequences for processes of exchange, reciprocity and justice. These issues are the focus of Chapter 3.

Chapter 3

Autonomy and togetherness

Issues of change in the family and marriage have been subject to discussion for many decades. These discussions have been characterised by worries and a sense of doom on the one hand, and of optimism and faith in the future on the other. Different eras have highlighted various 'problem areas' for discussion (Kollind 2002). Some present-day problem areas concern fragile bonds between spouses, as well as conflicts between freedom and togetherness. For example, Ulrich Beck and Elisabeth Beck-Gernsheim (1995) claim that our times are signified by 'a collision of interests between love, family and personal freedom', where the nuclear family, with its foundation in the different status of the genders, 'crumbles when addressed by issues of emancipation and equal rights, which no longer make a convenient halt outside our private lives' (Beck and Beck-Gernsheim 1995: 1–2). Personal interests and needs are confronted by needs of family ties; equal rights and issues of equality are confronted by the gender-based practices of family life. Fundamentally, these issues concern the tense relationship between autonomy and togetherness, between the 'I' and its aspirations towards a 'we' and its needs.

Every new couple is in one way or another confronted by issues regarding mine, yours and ours, but the ways of solving them are very far from being evident. Conflicts between personal and joint needs may arise in several different areas: money, contact with relatives and friends, leisure activities and managing household work. Safeguarding the togetherness is an important striving for most people, but to what costs, if it means compromising personal strivings and needs? When do personal demands undermine the prerequisites of together-ness? The purpose of this chapter is to shed light on issues of autonomy and togetherness in family relations, a theme that will remain with us throughout the book.

Let us first clarify that we refer to autonomy in a relative sense. No man is an island, as the seventeenth-century poet John Donne wrote, human kind does not exist outside a social context. What we understand as human is founded on and created through social relations. Autonomy can therefore only ever refer to a lesser grade of a constraint, or a larger space for the wishes or needs of the individual. In the context of this discussion, the question of autonomy is highly related to women's and men's different conditions. When women claim their personal freedom within the frame of the family ties, it carries a different meaning compared to the men, because family signifies different things to women and men.

The individualisation of love and family life

Autonomy as a concept was originally incorporated in a political and philosophical context, and belongs in the political process of democratisation. It is connected to the notion that individual rights should be the same for everybody, and be protected through contracts and rules (Benhabib 1992). Eventually, the concept became synonymous with independence, being economically and socially self-sufficient. The concept of autonomy is related to individualisation, the term given to the dynamic societal process that has led to fundamental transformations of economic, social, political and religious institutions. Market economy, political democracy and freedom of religion are examples of some of its consequences. The sociological connotation of individualisation is thus not equated with increased self-centredness. Instead, it concerns basic changes of social structures containing expansions of space for the individual to act independently of collective ties. These changes imply that the choices and life perspectives of the individual have now entered into the foreground. In other words, changes in working life, educational systems and standard of living have paved the way for the individual's freedom of choice. This freedom of choice applies to all choices, from choosing an education and profession to what emotional relationships one wants to enter. In this perspective, individualisation implies a development towards democracy and individual freedom.

The role of the family as a mediator of norms and traditions has lessened with this development, and the material motives for starting a family are no longer as relevant. The needs of the individual to be able to establish close social relationships remain, however, and needs for love, emotional closeness and trusting relationships are still important motives for starting families. While family life has become more geared towards emotional needs, the demands for quality in social relationships increase. More and more people choose to leave relationships that they perceive as destructive. Increasing divorce rates can be interpreted as a consequence of higher demands and expectations of what the marriage or relationship will provide in return. This is particularly the case for married women, who previously had to 'abandon their hopes if they were disappointed', but nowadays cling to their hopes and abandon the marriage (Beck and Beck-Gernsheim 1995: 62). In modernity, there are 'ethics of change' which also denote a striving towards optimising one's chances in life. With slight exaggeration, we can claim that social relationships have become interchangeable in a way that would have been unthinkable a mere few generations back.

The element of interchangeability is central in the new ideal of love that Giddens (1992) claims is developing. As opposed to previous ideals of love, it is not the person but the relationship which occupies the central position, and along with it the mutual exchange of intimacy and satisfaction that it may give. The perspective of this love relationship is not lifelong, but related to the exchange itself. So long as it is positive for both parties, the relationship is maintained, if it is not dissolved. The 'pure relationship' does not rest on any 'external' economic or material conditions, but is based on trust, communication and a mutual giving and taking. However, the conditions remain continuously unsure; the relationship is created as a 'rolling contract' (Giddens 1992: 192). The idea of the pure relationship underlines the ideal of the relative autonomy of both parties in a love relationship, which makes it different from a romantic love ideal.

According to Giddens, the new love ideal is part of the democratisation of our personal lives. Improved conditions for real autonomy are considered important for resisting and rejecting oppression in love relationships. Rules of negotiation and open communication are claimed to be important for enabling people to unleash their 'actions from an unconsciously organised power game' and create increased autonomy (Giddens 1992: 193). Autonomy, mutuality and satisfying exchange are thus regarded as prerequisites for equal love relationships.

Interpreting love and family relationships in terms of transactions is not a new phenomenon. A relatively large amount of research has been done on transactions between spouses, what values they exchange, and how power relations are created and maintained through asymmetries in the exchange. Several researchers use formulae in their understanding of family relationships, frameworks that include considerations of stakes, costs and returns. This is particularly accentuated in situations where the couple relations are dissolving, such as divorce (Moxnes 1990; Bloch et al. 1992). But also in a daily interaction, these factors apply. Kaufmann (1992) purports that family relationships are maintained through chains of 'gifts' and 'debts'. In a study on how spouses handle chores such as clothing maintenance and laundry, his claim is that there are two central 'economies' in a marital relation, i.e. the gift economy and the debt economy. 'Gift economy' implies that the spouses do not consciously calculate a gift in return when they carry out chores for each other. The overtly calculating approach is regarded as the opposite of what the marriage is expected to be – a mutual giving and taking in the name of love. Negotiations between partners are therefore made covertly. They do not want to openly acknowledge the actual stakes, costs and debts. 'Debt economy' is, however, made apparent in situations of perceived injustice. In such a case, open discussions about what you have given and received may become necessary. The notion of exchange, according to Kaufmann (1992), is an important aspect of the interaction between parties.

An even more articulated view of the family in terms of exchanges/transactions is provided by economic analyses made since the 1980s, where the relationships in the family are analysed on the same premises as businesses and economic systems. Numerous studies based on such presumptions have been made on a range of marital phenomena such as divorce, division of labour in the household and allocation of resources (for example, Bolin 1997). Yet even more subtle questions such as fidelity, love and care have been the subject of such analysis. The research that has come to characterise this field is the economist Gary Becker's (1993) analyses of the family in *A Treatise on the Family*. His discussion of the fundamentals of family togetherness and solidarity provides an example of an economic analysis of subtle questions.

An important point made by Becker is that the family and the market are favoured by different types of driving forces. The effective and good family is directed by altruistic actions, whereas egotism and self-interest are more effective in the market (Becker 1993: 299). The principle of equal allocation is representative of a type of altruism that is effective in the family, whereas distribution according to merit is more important in the market. If husband and wife divide the shares of consumption equally, it favours all family members. This principle of allocation in fact serves as insurance for every member of the household. Accidents and loss of income will not have as drastic consequences for the singular member of the household as in the case of allocation according to merit. Becker is particularly interested in what happens in a family group in which only one adult family member is altruistic, and the other is selfish. His thesis states that altruism breeds altruism in the family system. A selfish family member depends on the altruist's will and ability to give, and is therefore unable to make too high demands. Thus, the selfish family member will modify his/her demands and calculate the interests of the other.

Even if Becker makes a clear distinction between selfish and altruistic acts, his view of altruism is anchored in a utilitarian tradition that is connected to self-interest. Altruism governs when the 'utilitarian function' of one person depends on the well-being of another. When one person performs actions that are appreciated by another, this increases the utility of the person performing the action. Thus, altruistic actions become a way to increase one's self-interest (Becker 1993: 278–279). In the type of analysis made by Becker, the given starting point is that of the individual, whose actions are determined by the relative disadvantages and benefits that are generated by the alternative actions. Self-interest and calculations of benefit also direct the actions of the altruistic family members, although the utility is connected to welfare of the other person – not the self.

Becker has been criticised by feminists for not taking into account aspects such as oppression and unequal distribution of power, yet the theoretical perspective remains appealing. The systematic way in which self-interest and calculations of benefits and value occupy the central position in the analysis of the actual family has given rise to new approaches in the understanding of family life. This direction of research has also showed that families – not least in the unpaid labour of women – represent a substantial proportion of the economic activity and production of human capital in society.

This kind of economic analysis is representative of an intellectual tradition that to a large extent is characterised by the individualisation of society. The point of origin in this analysis, as mentioned above, is the individual, whose actions are attributed their rationale from the benefit calculations perspective. As we have seen, this orientation also identifies the individuals in the 'pure relationship' according to Giddens (1992) that necessitates a relatively autonomous individual.

Two approaches to the self and togetherness

Milton C. Regan (1999) has argued that the kind of tradition of economic analysis that Becker (1993) represents has a very particular approach to the self. Regan calls this the 'external stance', which refers to an approach that all people can apply when they observe themselves and the world around them, including love and family relationships. In order to gain a more independent way of evaluating our circumstances in life, we must create distance between ourselves and our attachments. Reflection on current circumstances requires an external point of comparison. Only then can we take a stand regarding the alternatives that we desire and the practical possibilities of choice. To reflect upon and question one's current circumstances in life implies mentally positioning oneself outside of them and then to differentiate and assume a more autonomous stance. The individual's own values, rather than a more general system of norms, must form the point of departure. The notion of justice, demand for agreement and a propensity for contractuality in the relationship are other aspects of what Regan (1999) considers to be the external stance. He states that this concept emphasises the notion that we are not shaped in any predetermined way, but that we can choose our goals and ask ourselves who we want to be.

Applied in private relationships, situations of family and love, the external stance can be regarded as an aspect of societal individualisation. Regan claims that it is this side of human thinking and acting that forms the basis of economic analyses, i.e. the relatively free and differentiated individual. However, the external stance is not the only or dominating stance. The 'internal stance' is equally important, dealing with attachment, social ties and togetherness; it represents another rationality.

Most people consider it to be important to create and maintain good, close and satisfying personal ties with other people. In relationships that are characterised by affection and generosity, there are also feelings of belonging. The ability to have relationships of this kind requires something other than distance and reflection on benefits and disadvantages. It requires a capacity to feel like a participant and part of a collective with other people. This is what Regan (1999) refers to in the expression 'internal stance'.

An important aspect of this stance is the ability to maintain personal attachments for their own sake, completely separate from considerations of costs and revenues. The existence of intimacy is taken for granted as providing meaning to life. In such an attachment, there is trust. It can also be based on an ongoing relationship, either in love or in something else, but is not preceded by choices, considerations or decisions. Unconditional trust, without questioning or evaluating, is a competence inherent in the internal stance.

Another important trait of this stance is the diffuse boundaries between the self and the other. Regan talks about the 'expanding self', a stance that implies neither egotism nor self-denial. This self includes the other in its identity. Being in love is normally seen as a case of obliterated boundaries. Persons who are in love tend to differentiate very little between the self and the other when it comes to sharing of resources. They take the perspective of the other, and are quick to ascribe attributes of the other to the self in a complex process of boundary-dissolving identification. Yet it is not only in love (or religious ecstasy) that this takes place. Individual identities are constituted in and through groups. This is exemplified by Berger and Kellner's (1970 [1964]) description of the identity transformation that is achieved through marriage, when two strangers gradually construct their jointly shared world. In daily conversations about the present, the past and the future, the separate biographies of the parties are transformed into a shared biography. In this reconstructed world, the spouses eventually create new images of themselves and the other (Berger and Kellner, 1970 [1964]). It can be difficult for the involved parties to overview this identity transformation, since it takes place in the unreflective circumstances that compose a vital framework for the social existence of humanity.

According to Regan (1999), external and internal stances constitute two different types of rationality. Attachment, identification with other people and the will to uphold close social relationships is not something that can be attributed to a fundamental, individualistic orientation, self-interest or similar. It is a different but equally basic human behavioural orientation.

The interview is an example of a situation that contributes to eliciting an external stance in the interviewee. When we were asking questions in our investigation about everyday life, division of labour and handling the economy, we forcefully extracted reflections and comparisons of various kinds. Yet following a conversation about laundry, household labour, money and children, other dimensions were occasionally included, one of them being love. For example, one woman said spontaneously, 'It is absolutely clear to me that he and I should live together, see. Forever.'

Such statements can be viewed as attempts to include central aspects of the relationship that were not included in the interview questions: they provide a showcase of what belongs in the internal stance.

The distinction made by Regan (1999) is not entirely new. The presumption that there are two entirely different types of stances in groups and individuals is the central theme of an early sociological train of thought. It is built into the concepts of sociability (*Gemeinschaft*) and society (*Gesellschaft*), as well as in the differentiation between primary and secondary groups, among other concepts. Another example is David Cheal (1988), who differs between political and moral economies in his study of the significance of gifts in modern society. The political economy interprets gifts in terms of social exchange and self-interest, and does not recognise alternative interpretations. The moral economy, on the other hand, considers relationships of trust and people's interest in reproducing lasting social relationships. Micro-worlds of basic social relationships are created in all social situations, because they provide predictability and safety for the lives of the involved. Love, care and affection are aspects of this (Cheal 1988). Similarly to Regan, Cheal maintains that there are two fundamentally different types of acts. When people give each other gifts, this act is sometimes incorporated in a moral economy situation, leading to the maintenance of social relationships. At other times, gifts are purely instrumental, leading to calculated, expected effects. One and the same individual is capable of both acts.

Four elementary types of human relationships

The social psychologist Allan P. Fiske (1991, 1992) has a similar interest for rationalities of action, but he differentiates four types of social relationships. Two of them are associated with what we discussed above, i.e. external and internal stances. Yet Fiske gives more attention to differentiating between types of relationships than does Regan (1999). In our opinion, Fiske's typology contributes to a deeper understanding of the relationship between autonomy and togetherness. One of the advantages of his typology is that it connects types of social relationships with different types of social exchanges and judgements of fairness.

Fiske sketches four elementary models used by people to create, understand, coordinate and evaluate social situations. The models do not specify how people should act in singular situations, but rather represent a set of rules that provide a certain framework to the existing repertoire of acts (Fiske 1991, 1992). According to Fiske, each person acquires these sets of rules during his/her upbringing, and they exist in all societies. We are not considering whether this claim is reasonable, we are merely using his theory in order to differentiate between different types of social relationships, i.e. forms of togetherness.

The model used by Fiske denotes that *communal sharing* is partly related to the internal stance, or moral economy. This is a type of relationship in which the group is superior in relation to the individuals. The self is highly integrated with the relationships within the group. Sameness is given priority over difference. The exchange is needs-oriented and has no clear boundaries between what is 'mine' and 'yours'; the terms are rather 'what is mine is yours'.

The type of relationship that Fiske calls *market pricing* is to some extent similar to the external stance. This relationship model, which we prefer to call *calculating*, is characterised by a high degree of independence among the individuals. This independence exists relative to the individuals and the togetherness which is created through their transactions. The exchange is in focus – the proportions of giving and taking. Negotiation, bargaining and making arrangements are typical ingredients in this kind of exchange. In this form of togetherness, it is the individual rather than the group that has a superior position.

The third type of relationship unifies aspects of both these models, without being reduced to either. It thus constitutes a distinct social relationship. Fiske refers to it as *equality matching*. Individuals in this relationship are oriented towards balance and reciprocity in the exchange. The principle of sameness is central. Each person expects to receive and contribute equal amounts. Exchanges are of the same kind, and cannot be transformed into other 'currencies'. If one party invites the other to dinner, the guest is expected to return the invitation – in due course. The dinner may be exchanged by something else, but not with money, in which case the party transcends an unwritten rule, thereby confounding the equality matching type with that of the calculating type. In equality matching, it is vital that each person has an equally strong voice. It is also vital that they have equal opportunities. Individuals in this type of relationship have a certain degree of autonomy in relation to one another.

There are some similarities between equality matching and what the sociologist Alvin Gouldner (1973) calls the norm of reciprocity. This norm stipulates, 'people should help those who have helped them' (Gouldner 1973: 242). Social relationships can be initiated by giving a gift, exchanging favours, or performing other acts that are perceived as valuable. The receiving party is 'tied' to the giving party. A feeling of gratitude is created along with an urge to reciprocate. The feeling of being indebted causes a will or obligation to reciprocate. The giving party will feel that sooner or later, something equal will be returned to him/her. The reciprocation can thus become the beginning of a new debt. In this way, loyalties and social bonds are created (Gouldner 1973; see also Simmel 1996 [1908]; Komter 1996). This norm incorporates an element of equality. However, the exchange may risk becoming lopsided, and the ensuing imbalance in the relationship causes one party to become superior, and the other 'indebted'. Power relationships then emerge, and the mechanisms are the same as those described in anthropological studies on gifts (Mauss 1972 [1925]).

The fourth relationship in Fiske's typology is, in fact, about power relationships and asymmetries between persons and group members. Hierarchies and rank orders are described in terms of gender, age, formal power, money, charisma, wisdom etc. Fiske refers to this as *authority ranking*. It is a formal power relationship based on consent. The principle of exchange is defined through the superiors agreeing with the subordinates, but the superiors have responsibilities to the subordinates in a paternalistic fashion. This model also requires loyalties between members, as well as the perception that the forms of allocation reflect justice.

A good illustration of these various models is provided by marriage, in the legal sense and in its changing form. Less than one hundred years ago, marriage was defined as an entity headed by the man, whose right it was to administer the finances of the woman, and represent her in legal issues. The marriage entity was considered as superior to the singular individuals, and the man was considered to be superior to the woman. Two relationship types were unified, that of authority ranking and communal sharing. The legal changes of the twentieth century meant that the married woman was given an independent position in the marriage. Both spouses had an equal say in financial and other issues from that point onwards, and a married woman could represent herself in legal matters. This change implied increased autonomy for the married woman. It can also be described as a shift in basic models of togetherness. Equality matching was now the norm, as opposed to authority ranking. Simultaneously, common sharing remained in terms of the spouses' responsibilities toward each other and their financial assets. However, settlements could also be made to avoid the latter, in accordance with the calculating model.

The law now regards husband and wife as independent individuals to a large extent. Each has their own property, money etc. Yet there are elements of joint sharing. An example of this asset combination is in the case of divorce, when assets are pooled, regarded as joint and divided equally, in principle.

The interweaving of models that per se represent different systems of norms naturally does not apply to only legal relationships. Equality is an ideal that shapes people's images of how a relationship should be nowadays. Equality is sought for in a number of different circumstances, along with certain independence in relation to the other. That which is included in common sharing – cohesion, care, safety and belonging – is equally important. Thus, togetherness occupies the central position, as opposed to independence. Hierarchical relationships between man and woman also remain, sometimes in ways that are not acknowledged. Authority ranking has not ceased to characterise family relations, despite the leaps made to promote equality. People try to manage several types of relationships in family and couple relationships, simultaneously or stepwise. Tensions are created by the fact that these relationship types are based on different conceptions of justice, rights and obligations, principles of allocation and moral judgement.

In couple relationships that are dominated by equality matching, justice is interpreted in terms of equality. Each person should have not only equal rights, but also equal obligations. Positive and negative things should preferably be allocated equally, and this principle of allocation is seen as just and fair. The following example of a line from everyday life illustrates this way of interpreting justice: 'Now that you have had the car all week, it is my turn to have it next week.' If the calculating orientation dominates, it may imply that the person with most resources will have more to spend on him or herself, and that justice is perceived in proportional terms. Using the car situation in another example from everyday life, this interpretation of justice would be: 'I will have the car most of the time, because I am the one paying for it.' When joint sharing is in the foreground, aspects of need take control. Obligations and rights are here based on specific situations, and are directed by mutuality in the consideration for both person's needs. Principles of allocation are primarily based on needs, and fairness is judged in terms of needs: 'You take the car, you're tired today. I'll take the bus.' In an authority ranking situation, one party has a secured right to certain things that are lacking the other party. Both parties can view differences in assets as unproblematic and fair. 'My husband uses the car a lot, and wants it to be available to him. And that's not so strange because cars are important to men. But he is nice and lets me use it every once in a while.'

It is possible that couples can choose only one model for their togetherness, but it is more probable that they construct their togetherness in a blend of models. This creates tensions between tendencies to act, different ways of viewing justice, between strive for autonomy and obligation. It also leads to very different perceptions and expressions of equality in the family life. As we will see, elements of these various relationship models are represented more or less evidently in the ways that couples reason about their everyday lives.

Obligations and rights in couple relationships

In the beginning of this chapter, we emphasised that individualisation has led to increased freedom of choice and that the patterns of duties and rights are not as clear as they were previously. We will briefly return to these questions in this section.

In a British study on obligations between kin, the authors highlight two types of norms of conduct (Finch 1989; Finch and Mason 1993). The first type states that close relatives who need help should be helped. This is a general norm regarding obligations, based on a person's position in a network of relatives. The second norm states that help and support for relatives is contextual and depends on the situation of the concerned parties. You help out the person that you have a positive relationship with. Loyalties and a sense of duty to support come in play here. In the absence of a positive relationship, there is no such feeling of duty to support, not even if the family relationship is close. Positive relationships are created through a mutual giving and taking (see also Gouldner 1973). Finch and Mason (1993) thus claim that people think and act towards kin in terms of norms regarding obligations based on position on one hand and mutuality on the other. These norms exist side by side and may strengthen or sometimes weaken each other.

There is an important distinction to be made between obligations based on position (or status) and mutuality respectively. The former are often specified. A certain position carries certain obligations. In marital relationships, gender has been the cornerstone in the system of rights and obligations. The rights of the man in the family have been regarded as e.g. coming home to a cooked meal; the woman's obligation has been to cook that meal. The man's obligation has been to earn money; the woman's right was to be supported. The obligations based on mutuality are considerably less specified; they are more variable and can be decided depending on the situation (Gouldner 1973).

A change in the marital relationship, regardless of whether the parties are married or cohabiting, is that gender-based obligations no longer have the same legitimacy. It is no longer taken for granted that the woman does the cooking and the man earns the money. Even if many women still have the main responsibility for the household, it cannot be taken for granted. Although such gender-based norms still influence people's thinking and acting, they are seen as problematic and controversial. People cannot assume that only one way of acting is the right way. An example of this is how couples discuss parental leave. Some couples think it is a matter of course that the woman stays at home with the child during the entire period. It is regarded as a woman's right or obligation, depending on how one chooses to see it. Others share the time unquestioningly. It is something both of them should do and be part of. The issue may still be controversial to others, who have different views on how the time should be shared. For instance, the man may want more time in parental leave than the woman is willing to give him (Kugelberg 1999; Plantin 2001). The rights and obligations of women and men concerning the small child are not fixed.

The fact that norms concerning gender-based obligations are controversial implies that such norms are not easily given open acknowledgement. Instead of justifying a choice of action for reasons based on gender, it is motivated in other ways, using different arguments.

Obligations determined by gender constitute part of a type of social relationship that is characterised by authority ranking and hierarchy, in Fiske's (1991, 1992) terminology. Obligations derived from reciprocity, on the other hand, are developed in other types of social relationships. In the cases where an equal balance is sought for, there is a striving towards creating a balance of obligations and rights. In social relationships that are signified by a communal sharing, the aim is primarily to satisfy the jointly shared needs of the group. Also in the calculating social relationship, systems of obligations and rights are formulated. These are chiefly based on agreements that in turn rely on what you give and what you receive. In all relationship types where obligations and rights are not based on a position such as age or gender, there is scope for variation and a certain level of unpredictability. The fact that gender-based obligations and rights no longer are taken for granted is an important reason for the increase in space to manoeuvre and negotiate in families. As was mentioned previously, negotiations are regarded as an important part of modern family life. In Chapter 4, we will discuss acts of negotiation in couple relationships and further touch upon issues of autonomy and togetherness.

Chapter 4

Negotiations, conditions and strategies

In the previous chapter, we maintained that views on justice are related to the specific social circumstances in which justice is evaluated. The relationship model that individuals follow bears consequences for how justice or injustice is evaluated, or for what is regarded as morally right or wrong.

In this chapter, we will discuss different ethical positions on allocation of resources, labour and togetherness. We will also present our view on negotiations and the various dimensions therein, such as power, gender and needs. The purpose is to provide a more in-depth understanding of patterns according to which couples manage conflicts between the self and togetherness, autonomy and dependence, as well as for how equality is perceived.

Family culture and ethical principles

The Swiss sociologist Kellerhals and colleagues (1988, 1997), like Fiske (1991, 1992), claim that principles of justice vary according to what type of togetherness or group cohesion is strived for. Thus, principles of justice are not founded in rigid preconceptions of justice, but formulated in specific situations. Kellerhals assumes that family cohesion expresses itself in different family styles or cultures, as we prefer to call them. With the purpose of classifying different family cultures, he uses three dimensions – principles of cohesion, integration and regulation.

Group *cohesion* is characterised by dimensions of individualism and collectivism respectively. On one end of the spectrum, we can imagine a group consisting of independent and individualistic individuals, perceiving themselves as different to one another, with separate interests, activities, attitudes and tastes. On the other end, the individuals are alike and perceive themselves in a state of 'fusion'. Emphasis in this case is on consensus and group unity in relation to its surroundings. Interests and values are shared, and there is a strong notion of 'our family'. Group *integration* denotes its degree of closeness or openness towards the surroundings. On one extreme, openness towards the surroundings appears to be a condition for survival. The other extreme is characterised by suspicion and disbelief of others who do not belong to the family, a self-sufficient 'my home is my castle'. *Regulation* concerns how the individuals in a family coordinate their actions and relationships. On one extreme, the relationships are rule-bound and follow clear normative patterns. On the other end of the spectrum, the joint actions follow a freer pattern of communication, where discussions are held and arguments, explanations and negotiations are made.

These three dimensions are combined to form family cultures. For example, one can imagine a family where both parents work full time in professions that are career oriented, with high demands on commitment in work-related activities outside the regular working hours. Work-related guests are often received in the home, and one of the parents is often away on business journeys. The family tempo is high, message notes and instructions are written for family members. The outward communication is on a high level, whereas internally, communication is low. Steadfast rules for interaction are not maintained, but are determined situationally. The opposite of this family culture is one where all family members meet regularly, and there are many shared activities. The family interacts mainly in its own sphere, and outings are made together. Meticulous records are kept on who gets what, and the degree of fairness regarding allocation of resources is often a subject in family discussions. Justice is decided through arguments on needs. In this case, it is important to point out that a certain type of family culture is based on specific action strategies that work to uphold the family culture itself. This means that these kinds of families create their own rationality regarding that which is perceived as just and fair; we can call this family-based principle of justice.

From the empirical research that Kellerhals et al. (1988, 1997) have conducted, it emerges that the types of cohesion and arguments that the families make regarding justice vary according to social class. Family cohesion in lower social classes tends to emphasise the superiority of the group identity rather than the individual's. Agreements tend to be normative rather than communicative. This implies that one identifies the rule systems that will govern rather than creating the order through discussions. The emphasised logics of justice are based on rank, status and property as opposed to contributions, such as efforts made and resources. The needs and demands of family members matter more than cost and benefit thinking. Cohesion in families of a higher social class is instead characterised by its emphasis on the independence and individuality of the individuals. Negotiations tend to be openly communicative. Cost and benefit calculations are of greater importance. The principles of justice applied accentuate either a contractual approach or contextual judgement, i.e. determination by circumstance and situation. Furthermore, external criteria are often used to judge actions. Efforts made by singular persons are judged according to individual circumstances. Status and categorical reasoning have a smaller place when judging efforts made by the individual (Kellerhals et al. 1988).

The togetherness in a family circle thus consists of locating a convenient boundary between individuality and dependence. A very low degree of cohesion and integration makes it difficult to uphold a group formation in the first place, whereas high levels of cohesion and integration provide limited space for the individual. In his studies, Kellerhals also found that women and men have different views on family togetherness and values of justice. The women were more inclined to think about the best interests of the group, whereas men were more inclined towards individual needs. Gender differences in ethical approaches have been a hot topic for discussion for many years.

Justice and relationship ethics in social togetherness

The relationship between individual needs and needs of togetherness are central themes in Carol Gilligan's (1982, 1988) research on ethical and social matura-tion from a gender perspective. She differentiates between two moral perspec-tives, *justice* and *care*. These ethical perspectives or moral orientations concern the judgement of relationships – not only what is regarded as important, but also how one views oneself in relationships. Justice orientation means that relationships are judged in terms of equal values that are balanced on scales or degrees of equality. In the justice perspective, oppression and inequality are perceived as moral problems that one attempts to solve. Care ethics entail a striving to care for others, being responsive to the problems and needs of others. From the care ethics perspective, distance and abandonment are regarded as morally opposed to attentiveness and responsiveness. In care ethics, dissociation and abandonment are regarded as part of a moral stance that is contrasted by attentiveness and responsiveness. On the basis of several empirical studies, Gilligan draws the conclusion that all relationships contain both types of moral considerations, but in most cases, one of the principles dominates over the other. The claim she makes based on her empirical work is that women to a higher degree utilise the care ethics in decision-making situations, whereas men utilise the justice perspective. However, the difference between the genders is not sharp. Gilligan (1982) stresses that both perspectives host two ways of reasoning in relationships, that it is a matter of themes rather than gender.

The research pursued by Gilligan and associates has been subjected to count-less discussions and reflections in works of philosophy, psychology and social science that focus on gender. The terminology in these has varied – rights ethics, logics of justice, care ethics have been featured, to mention a few. Gilligan her-self uses the terms 'justice' and 'care' to distinguish moral orientations, but does not discuss principles of justice. We prefer the term 'relationship ethics' to care ethics, in order to avoid associations to 'care' or 'care work', which constitute factors in a special type of relationship.[1] In the following section, we give an in-depth presentation of the differences between the various moral orientations applied to families.

Justice and relationship ethics on a family level

Justice can have many different meanings. For example, justice can be understood in terms of having achieved similar results regardless of the amount of input, such as equal child allowance for all. Justice can also be related to effort, i.e. it is fair that you get out the equivalent to what you put in. In this case, child allowance would increase in proportion to how many children a person gives birth to. The more children, the greater the allowance. A third notion of justice is associated with needs: what you are given is in accordance with your needs. Needs-tested child allowance is an example of this. Clark and Chrisman (1995) argue that close relationships are strongly dominated by needs-oriented justice. Needs-based principles of justice, however, are not maintained in relationships at all costs, according to Clark and Chrisman. Depending on specific circumstances, certain situations can be perceived as transcending a symbolic limit where this rule no longer applies.

Needs-based justice is not the same as relationship ethics, because this type of ethics is not associated with justice as a principle of allocation. Relational ethics entails being attentive and responsive to others and the self. Yet, individuals relate to both justice and relational ethics in social togetherness.

Ethics of justice originate from the independence and freedom of the individual. Justice thus represents ethics where the individual's autonomy and resources for freedom of choice are emphasised. Relational ethics are more focused on mutual dependence and responsibility for others. Justice ethics and relational ethics are not principally opposed, and in everyday interaction, the individual applies both principles (Gilligan 1988; Gilligan and Attanucci 1988). The issue is rather which ethical perspective is the dominant in social negotiations. With justice ethics as the guiding principle, letting the involved parties voice their interests and mediate allocations that are felt as reasonable and legitimate can create togetherness. Allocations based on principles of justice in social togetherness can be taken quite far without causing splits, on the condition that all parties remain confident that their agreements also apply in practice. When the results of the negotiations are viewed as legitimate and right, and are followed up in practice, togetherness is created that builds on trust, openness and respect.

The various principles of ethics contain different views of the self in relation to others in the context of social togetherness. From a justice perspective, the self is seen as autonomous and capable of differentiating from others. Here lies a striving towards impartiality and objectivity in relation to others. The self is protected by rules and contracts for collaboration. The autonomous self views others in terms of self-mirroring or self-reflection. Others become a means to discover or acknowledge the self, with boundaries between 'me' and 'you'.

From the perspective of relational ethics, the self is described as 'connected'. The significance of this is human engagement, responsiveness and interactivity, and that the individual recognises the needs of others based on their situation.

The self is seen as flowing between the individual and others. In this perspective, morals means attending to the needs of others, seeing and caring for them, alleviating their problems and listening to them. In this case, interdependence is more important than independence. The self is transformed through the experience of deeper contacts with others. However, the perception of the self in interaction with others needs to be clarified further.

Because relational ethics imply responsiveness to the needs of others, Gilligan (1988) draws attention to the risk of diffusing the needs of the self with that of others. Attention directed at others may, however, also result in the individual caring for him/herself by also caring for others (Gilligan 1988). This is an act of balance between perception of the self and its needs and terms on the one hand, and on the other hand, the needs and conditions of others. These needs and terms can either be regarded as flowing from obligations and rights in relation to the positions of wife and husband, or they can be regarded as a reflection of their own personal terms – for example, in cases where the element of obligations is not integrated in the perception of self. Gilligan uses the term 'commitment', an agreement to carry out something for someone, a connection with emotional and moral impetus. Gilligan differs between two kinds of commitments, the *duty commitment* and the *relational commitment*. Duty commitment corresponds to status-based obligations/rights. It may also entail shouldering a responsibility and sticking to it, as a kind of contract that it is one's duty to fulfil. Relational commitment is better understood in terms of 'being responsive'. It means that the individual takes the initiative to get to know the needs or problems of others, and respond to the perception of these. The issue at stake here is to listen to the other, but also to be aware of your own needs and be prepared to find a solution that involves both parties. Actions are viewed in the light of mutual responsibility and dependence founded in a system of reciprocity.

In Figure 1, which is based on Attanucci (1988), we attempt to make this reasoning visual in four different ways of approaching the needs of the self and others.

Figure 1 Relationships on whose terms – the individual's perspective on self and others

		Perspectives on the self	
		OBLIGATIONS	ON OWN TERMS
Perspectives on the other	OBLIGATIONS	Governed	Self-oriented
	OWN TERMS	Altruistic	Mutual

1 In the *governed* case, perspectives on the self and the other are governed by obligations and family norms. Such a relationship is fairly stereotyped, without much need to communicate about rights and duties.

2 In the *altruistic* case, the woman sees herself as being governed by obligations and the other's terms have precedence over her own. This is a 'classical' case where the woman's needs have small scope: the self-needs. Her loyalty is based on conceptions of duty and she seldom regards her own needs as justified – they have to be subordinated to joint needs.

3 As a contrast we have the *self-oriented* attitude, where one's own wishes and needs take precedence over those of others whose needs and terms are perceived stereotypically.

4 The *mutual* case, where the needs and wishes of both the self and the other are considered, implies an active attitude, which relates one's own needs and wishes to those of the other. The main point in this mutual kind of attitude within a relationship is that the individual woman is able to take care of herself while also taking care of the other.

Negotiations

In creating a picture of how the participating couples display their divisions of household labour and childcare and make agreements on expenditure and consumption patterns, we have assumed that the responses given by the interviewees have been preceded by negotiations. The methodology of our study does not leave space for studying the negotiation process itself. However, we have been able to observe how the parties subsequently construct arguments and motivations for how the decisions were reached. In some cases, we were told that the negotiations have been explicit, bordering on conflicts. In everyday interaction, negotiations are usually hidden and implicit – a certain order has become operational without anyone shedding much thought on why. Relationships in the family also change over time, for example when children switch from pre-school to after-school care, change of jobs, onset of a new stage of education, redundancy, illness and so forth. Such events can lead to breaks in the life course, which give rise to reflection and questioning of the given order. Our questions have prompted the interviewees to think about their own motives for their allocation, partly based on an understanding of the partner's motives, and partly based on changes and reflections of changes.

With the aid of the theoretical perspectives that we have presented in this and Chapters 2 and 3, we have interpreted the arguments and motives of implicit and explicit negotiations regarding division of labour, money and influence of the interviewed couples. The purpose has been to study the influence that each party attributes to him/herself in decisions that concern both individual issues and jointly shared interests.

What do we mean by negotiation? We perceive it as a technique for handling opposing interests or aims. Negotiations are a way of resolving conflicts and gaining influence over decisions. Klein and White (1996) define negotiations as both parties stating their aims, and using their resources to convince the other party to move towards these respective aims. This view of negotiations implies the usage of communication and cooperation. Negotiation as conflict solving therefore differs from coercion and violence, which do not entail cooperation. This means that negotiations revolve around giving and taking in a process of exchange.

According to Thylefors (1996), conflict research assumes that individuals apply patterns of conflict that are individual and triggered by different types of situations in a largely similar way. Based on this assumption, five different strategies of conflict management emerge. Strategy is here referred to as an overarching approach towards interest and needs of the self and others.[2] If the individual's consideration for his or her own interests and that of others is combined with the greater scope of consideration for the interests of others, five combinations are elicited – competitive, cooperative, adaptive, avoiding and compromising. The competitive style involves great consideration for one's own interests, and little consideration of others' interests. The cooperative style entails great consideration for both own and others' interests. If an adaptive style is applied, this means great consideration for the interests of others, and a small amount of consideration for the own interests. The avoiding style entails a small amount of consideration to the interests of either, whereas the compromising style means sacrificing the needs of the self on the presumption that both parties will make sacrifices to their aims. One problem with this model is that it is based on the individual, and the styles described are also individual. According to Thylefors (1996), however, the styles are also descriptive of the quality of the relationship. The assumption is made that both individuals will develop a shared style – both competing, both cooperating, both compromising. Issues arise when the parties do not develop shared strategies, for example if one party competes while the other avoids. If in theory, the five individual styles were to be combined, twenty-five possible combinations would result. However, in negotiations, individuals have a tendency to adapt their strategies to one another, further underlining that conflict management is a process.

With inspiration from these models, we are presenting a typology for conflict management in negotiations based on relationships between two parties and their focus on their own needs in negotiations, as described in Figure 2.

In cases where both parties pursue their own needs and interests, the negotiations (at least initially) will be characterised by *competition* which means that both parties try to maximise their advantage in the negotiation. When both parties are prepared to emphasise their own needs less, they can also lessen their demands and achieve *compromise*. This combination may also lead to *avoidance* of the negotiations. Communication is avoided and subsequently also the reflection of one's needs and interests.

Subordination takes place when either party disregards his/her own needs, and focuses only on the satisfaction of the needs and interests of the other.

Figure 2 Styles of conflict management

		Focus on own needs, interests	
		High	Low
Focus on own needs, interests	High	Competition	Subordination
	Low	Subordination	Compromise or avoidance
Cooperation: Both safeguarding own and others' interests			

Subordination, like avoidance, can be regarded as fear of articulating one's needs, an expression of anxiety connected to the prospect of having to take a stand and choose. Thylefors (1996: 35) writes, 'conflicts clarify who I am – to myself'. This means that the conflict entails a challenge not only to the self and the self-image, but also to the dependence or independence of the individual. In this context, the individual's perspectives of the self and others respectively assume an important role in negotiations. For instance, if a person perceives him/herself as being obliged towards others, and that these obligations constitute the rights of others, it does not leave room for much negotiation. If one's own needs are perceived as negotiable in relation to the needs of others, the latter also being perceived as negotiable, the room for both negotiation and conflict is considerably larger.

On the one hand, individuals take into consideration their own needs or interests regarding the issue at hand in conflicts or negotiations, such as who is going to deal with the dishes. On the other hand, they also consider the wish to maintain the relationship, to remain friends and not get upset with one another (Thylefors 1996). In many cases, the issue at hand can be seen as symbolic for the togetherness. The model described in Figure 2 looks only to the issue at hand in the relationship. However, the motives to subordinate one's interests to the issue at hand can be interpreted as prioritising the relationship. For example, a quarrel about cleaning can create a bad atmosphere in the home. In order to avoid that, one party refrains from achieving a solution to the disagreement and ceases to argue, and the problem remains unsolved.

Another way of managing conflicts is to reach an acceptable solution through *cooperation*. In this situation, both parties assume that they have a shared problem that they will solve together. This necessitates the ability to communicate and listen, in order to understand the other and oneself. Negotiations strive towards penetrating the disagreements, and finding a solution that can satisfy both individuals' needs (Ekstam 2000). For example, a conflict about cleaning is put against the bigger picture, in which the couple make connections to other problems and interests. A more comprehensive analysis of the cleaning, work hours, pleasure and displeasure makes way for a solution that feels reasonable from both parties' perspectives.

Conflicts, power and influence

All negotiations derive from conflict. What 'conflict' really means in this context is naturally a matter of discussion. One definition of conflict that we have found to be fruitful is 'confrontation between individuals, or groups, over scarce resources, controversial means, incompatible goals, or combinations of these' (Sprey 1979: 134). Sprey's view of conflicts emphasises that it is a *process* rather than a condition, which signifies that conflicts are seen as related to underlying structures, such as gender conflicts. Conflicts can also be understood in terms of basic, conditional inequalities, and assume expression in concrete situations where these surface. Discontent with the division of labour in the household can be seen as an expression of women subordination to a male power, which is disengaged from the shared labour. The conflicts are not necessarily open or expressed in disputes. They can be hidden, and latently expressed in non-verbalised discontent, which at times will rise up to the surface (Ahrne and Roman 1997; Roman 1999). In subsequent chapters, we shall show how this takes shape in couple relationships, by presenting our results on couple negotiations concerning division of labour, money and influence.

Normative perceptions of gender constitute an 'impersonal' or tacit power that is personified in the negotiations that take place on an everyday level. We call this kind of power *normative power*. These normative perceptions are inherent in social institutions, and permeate human thoughts about needs and conditions of the self and of others from a gender perspective. This takes place both on the level of society and the family. When men and women in families negotiate with each other about how they should organise everyday life, it is not only a matter of economic or practical sense, but also a matter of creating an order that is compatible with subjective perceptions of masculinity and femininity, or rather how men and women ought to prioritise. This is illustrated by a study of men with managing positions in families where their careers had been made at the same time as they had small children. These men had a very strong work orientation, and their priorities as well as their self-image had been affirmed in terms of the support given to them by a mentor or a strong career role model. Their work orientation had become very strong, and was integrated with their identity perception. This implied that their loyalties and will to oblige towards work had become solidified in their self-perception. Work was given top priority and was also associated with the male identity of the breadwinning husband and father. In the study, it was said that the women's priorities were focused on the needs of the children, although they continued to work and maintained a strong professional identity. Regardless of their strategic professional choices, their actions were adaptable in regards to the family, children and husband to a much higher extent than that of the men. The women developed a priority order so that they could combine work and care tasks (Andersson 1993). Similar results and explanations are presented in other Swedish studies of couple relationships

(Ahrne and Roman 1997; Bäck-Wiklund and Bergesten 1997; Magnusson 1998; Roman 1999; Plantin 2001; Nyman 2002.) In these negotiations held by the couples, such as regarding who should take parental leave, there were arguments partly supportive of the subjective perceptions of the genders, and partly adaptive to structural circumstances beneficial to men, which were perceived as beneficial to the common good. Parental insurance objectively provides a good opportunity to share parental leave, but despite this, it was interpreted in the short run as being most economically advantageous, career-wise, and practically beneficial if mothers took the lion's share of the leave. The couples also said that this choice was most compatible with their values. Choices and priorities were made within a framework of expectations of their own and of their social surroundings, including employers. Employers do not in principle encourage men to take parental leave (Hwang 2000). In the general policy, both genders are encouraged to choose, but their choices are based on conditions that in the end make them traditional. The structures of expectations that regulate the negotiations of the couples form a normative power that acts through a series of complicated mechanisms.

Haavind (1987) provides an in-depth picture of how these norms act. She claims that women have chosen to fight subordination by expanding their options and to take control of their own lives. Women make themselves responsible for how they have utilised their possibilities. Failures are perceived as personal, since the choice is personal. As a consequence of the expanded options, Haavind maintains that female subordination has changed its direction or shape. According to Haavind, since women have adopted a more responsible and independent life in relation to themselves, men have been able to use this to free themselves from economic and emotional responsibility. When women assume the responsibility to make sure that everybody in the family (particularly the children) are fine, they may risk ending up in a spiral of demands of good housekeeping and for providing the best possibilities for the children – demands that are perpetuated in the media, in advertisements and in documentary programmes. These notions act as normative guidelines, and are more or less negotiable in the concrete relationship. However, it is based on the idea that women have the chief responsibility for the home and the children. This means that they will carry the blame if they cannot live up to the levels of ambition – whether they belong to themselves, the husband or the remaining surroundings. While women have the chief responsibility for the well-being of others in the family, they have limited control over the conditions that create this reality. Others dictate the needs that the woman must adjust to. Being adaptive and letting the needs of others take charge is central to the female stance. Ylva Elwin-Nowak (1999), in her book on guilt in modern motherhood, shows that mothers' responsibility for the children is based on being accessible and maintaining closeness. These notions are rooted in developmental theories that stress the importance of the early attachments between the mother and child. The aims therein create guiding influence on the adaptations made by women in everyday life in order to avoid feelings of inadequacy resulting from being unable to live up to them.

Different uses of power are thus central in the understanding of how conflicts are managed, that is how each person seeks to influence decisions. Power can also be *control over and possibility to influence others* but simultaneously *the ability of a person to make decisions in accordance with his/her aims*. This definition of power describes the exertion of control over others, i.e. a person's ability to impose his/her will despite resistance from others. Power involves not only having control and being able to influence others, but also being able to make decisions according to one's own goals. This definition implies that power is the capacity to make others do what they would not do on their own will. In this sense power is understood as control of others and a capacity to govern other people's behaviour. A second implication is that power can be understood as 'power over self' or 'self-governance', where the individual is able to make decisions without being constrained by a lack of alternatives, or is able to get their own way despite the opposition of others (Watts, 1991; Thagaard 1996). This is Thagaard's (1996) definition of *personal power*. In close relationships, dependencies of others and their conditions are always present. By highlighting self-governance, which is the possibility to make independent choices, priorities are brought into focus, i.e. own interests and the needs of others. By prioritising the needs of others, control can be gained in the togetherness. In this view, by making choices that prioritise the needs of others, a person does not surrender his/her influence as a matter of course. This is linked together with the aims underlying the choice. It is hence important to differentiate between the individual's strive to gain influence over their own situation, the needs of others or the common good.

In summary: power resources are central in negotiations. Power rests with various resources, money and income being the most important (Blumberg 1991; Chafetz 1991; Fenstermacher et al. 1991). Power that is connected to emotions and dependencies, and control over emotional needs and sexuality, are expressions of *emotional power*. Status is another resource of power, which we have tied to normative guidelines for the genders. The extent to which authority depends on gender, i.e. particular benefits claimed by the gender, is questioned and subject to attempts at transcending. It is interesting to study what factors are important in the balance between reciprocity and exchange in the negotiations held by the spouses. We are thus particularly interested in how gender boundaries are transcended and the arguments that occur therein. We are partly interested in the 'currencies' or values being exchanged, and partly in the importance of justice thinking relative to the relational ethics that apply. Lines of reasoning concerning what is morally right or fair are entrenched in the social dynamics of the family, and the type of social togetherness that forms a ruling principle in the family. The idea is that the social togetherness in the family is reproduced or recreated with the aid of various exchanges, and is thus connected to an understanding of what is morally right. The space given to individuals in these negotiations is of particular interest.

Conflicts may be hidden and expressed as non-verbalised discontent (Ahrne and Roman 1997). In the following chapters, we will outline the shape assumed by this discontent in different couple relationships, and describe how couples negotiate division of labour, money and influence.

Chapter 5

Division of labour in the household

Ideals, influence and conflicts

In our investigation of 1992, parents were asked about conflicts regarding household work. Only a small percentage said that these occurred everyday, whereas slightly more than one-third of the women and a scarce quarter of the men said these occurred sometime every week.[1] A majority of the interviewees – more than two-thirds – reported that such conflicts occurred never or rarely.

In the follow-up interview study of 1997, five years had passed. Life conditions of most of these men and women had changed – the children were now at school and life with small children was nothing but a memory. The investigation and interview methods themselves had also changed. At this point, the women and men were asked to describe the division of labour in the home: who does what, any conflicts and whether they perceived the division to be fair. Stories of conflicts were told as part of a relatively comprehensive description of everyday life in the family.

As in the previous study, roughly two-thirds reported relatively few conflicts regarding household work. In the other cases, the conflicts had more of a regular occurrence. However, conflicts can have very different characters. They can be highly tense, harsh words can be exchanged and be experienced as very destructive. They can also be experienced as a positive part of the interaction, an inescapable part of an open, argumentative lifestyle. Conflicts can also be like sour-dough, brewing and puffing without bursting or changing. Some of the couples, who claimed that their conflicts regarding household work were very rare, had a division of labour that we as outsiders judged to be clearly unfair. The absence of conflicts regarding household labour can thus not be taken as a sign that the division is fair.

We spoke with women and men about their division of labour. We asked what it looks like, why it has that appearance and if it is perceived as fair or unfair. Descriptions of what is done are naturally an ambiguous measure compared to practical reality. However, we assume that there is a certain connection between the couples' descriptions of their everyday life and its actual praxis. In cases of recurring routines that undeniably constitute a large part of household labour, much is taken for granted without reflection. That which is taken for granted is often hard to describe. The use of vignettes in the investigation was a method of bringing attention to the ordinary and daily. Additionally, there is the problem of social desirability – the wish to come across in a positive light in front of others. We cannot confidently say what the interviewees have chosen to exclude and under- or overemphasise in their stories. Yet, a picture of thinking and arguments surrounding issues of household labour can be extracted. Here it emerges what the interviewees considered to be of differing importance, and why they considered one type of division to be fair compared to another.

Here and in Chapter 6, we will deal with questions about norms and ideals that are applied in the sharing of household labour. Earlier we made the claim that nowadays, couples cannot reasonably avoid discourses on gender equality. Yet, we have also maintained that it is by no means clear what equality means in the family circumstance. Those who endorse the equality ideal must try with their partner to give it a meaning, and through concrete action also give it a practical significance. The sceptic and those who reject the ideal must still relate to it. He or she must formulate a division of labour that can be considered as good, in spite of the fact that it diverges from the equality ideal. This chapter will provide examples of how couples create a 'good' division of labour, and highlight the consequences, strategies and conflicts arising from this issue. This chapter presents various ways of organising household labour, and Chapter 6 describes the principles used to judge the degree of fairness or equality therein.

We open the chapter with a few examples of what characterises contented and discontented couples, and then move on to describe different ways of organising divisions of labour. The focus remains with the division of labour. When couples are referred to as discontented or contented, it is referred to only in this context, not in terms of the relationship as a whole or other aspects of the relationship.

Contented and discontented couples

> I think I do at least 75 per cent of the work. If you ask my husband, he won't think so at all. He thinks we do as much, but I don't think so. And we bicker a lot about it. It's as if in some way it is natural that I am the one always supposed to know what is in the fridge and freezer and be able to fix our meals.

This is the expression of a woman who is not altogether happy with the division of labour that has been established between her and her husband. Another woman who is responsible for almost everything in the home says that she detests household work: 'Yuck, it is disgusting, I hate cooking, I don't want to do the laundry, and I don't want to clean.' Yet, she is the one who does all of it. These are two examples of how women express their discontent with the division of labour in the household. Men also express discontent, albeit differently from the women. For example, one man expressed awareness of the heavier burden of his wife, saying that he 'should do more household chores'. Another man knows that his wife in fact 'carries too heavy a load in the house' and 'it gives me a guilty conscience, but it is hard to keep up. It wears on me, of course.' Some male interviewees gave the impression that they were uncomfortable discussing issues of household labour (which may have been heightened by the fact that the interviewer was a woman). Women who are discontented direct their irritation at the chores, their men or at themselves for taking on things that they should not take on. Men are more defensive and worry about handling the guilt conscience triggered by the woman's irritation.

Contented men and women think that their division of labour is fair and works for them. There is no need to argue about it, and it seldom affects the relationship negatively. 'I would think it terribly tiresome to argue about division of everything,' one woman commented, claiming that she never had to have such arguments.

So what type of division of labour are women and men discontented or content with? What does it look like and how did it come about? First, we can confirm that 'contented' couples can organise household labour in very different ways. There are couples where the woman manages the greater part of the household labour and views it as her area of responsibility – representing a high degree of traditional division of labour. There are also couples who have developed a cooperative style, where both are active in the household labour. Some couples used to quarrel regularly about the household labour at an earlier stage, but were eventually able to create a model that was satisfactory to both parties. In these cases, the women were the instigators of this change.

In some couples, it was clear that the woman had played a significant role in changing the division of labour in the household. Women in these cases come across as governing. Based on the issue of influence over household labour, two general types of couples can be discerned. In the first type, one party – the woman or the man – governs the organisation of household labour in a direction that is not perceived as a matter of course by the other party. For example, one party may demand that both of them should carry out equal amounts of the household labour, something that may not be fully acceptable to the other party. When one party wishes to have a certain division of labour that is not entirely acceptable to the other, it may constitute a potential basis for conflict in the couple relationship. Two expressed wills pull in different directions. The wills may not even be explicit, but rather expressed in terms of diffuse expectations or divergent states of alert. In the following sections, this type of couple will be categorised as 'one party governs' or making an attempt to direct.

In the second type of couple, no such active direction exists. Instead, a kind of jointly shared value system shapes the creation of the division of labour. The parties have the same, basic expectations. Nobody tries to actively steer the other party in a direction that is not a given to him or her. We refer to this broad category as 'both parties govern', but it could also be referred to as 'nobody governs'.

In couples where 'one party governs', both, one or none of the parties may be satisfied with the situation. This is also true of the other general category, in which 'both parties govern'. In the following section, we will provide examples and discuss such variations of directing and satisfaction. The purpose is not to promote a new typology of division of labour that categorises equality or lack of equality. Rather, it should be viewed as an attempt to highlight variations in the existing patterns.

One party governs

Successful female governance

In some couples, it appears that the women have made efforts to engage their men actively in household work, and they were successful in this endeavour. One woman says that she and her husband now have equality in their couple relationship, but that it hasn't always been that way. It has been a struggle:

> Well, I don't think we were equal to begin with, you know. Partly with cleaning and things like that, from the beginning I had to fight for us to become equal. But in the end, we were. And when the first child was young, I was the one who took care of him very, very much. And that led to trouble. He was with the childminder and it didn't work out and so we had to have him at home and there was a real battle about working hours . . . but now I don't think it's like that anymore. Now I think it works.

Reaching a better balance between the work hours of the spouses took fifteen years, according to this woman. During these years, there were plenty of fights. We are not told about her method, but she presents herself as a woman who made demands, did not capitulate or accept that the division of labour was not working. The message she brings across is that her stubborn struggle has finally been fruitful. The significance of the children's increasing independence over time is not mentioned.

In another couple, it is predominantly the husband who underlines the wife's struggle to make him do half of the work:

> And she has driven a very hard bargain. She says, if I had married someone more servile, I would have been lying on the sofa with the papers instead.

According to him, the wife has 'looked out for her own interests'. He also points out that she is quick to express herself in no uncertain terms when she sees that something is not working. It is not only a matter of 'doing your bit', but also that he is expected to conform to the norms that prescribe her order. According to his description, he is the one who has had to adapt to her norms, rather than the other way around. This is expressed in the following quote:

Somebody [the wife] makes demands, somebody has been making the decisions and said that we have to cope with this and I thought 'but is that
really necessary'. So I have pulled and she has pushed, and you have ended
up somewhere – surely to her advantage or closer to her norms but maybe
not entirely in the end.

The changes described by the couples above have taken place over a long period
of time, and led to fights and quarrels, discussions and deliberations, unfulfilled
promises and renewed conflicts. The change that the women have tried to bring
about has of course taken place interactively with the husband in a series of
conflicts, negotiations and concessions concerning the many routines of everyday life. Both the women and men in these couples are anxious to point out that
eventually, they did create a satisfying division of labour. The men are, however,
also anxious to point out that there are limits to the women's control.
Statements made in the following style illustrate this: 'I will go this far but not
further'; 'I agree to some things but not to that'. The concessions have their
limits, which will also be exemplified below.

There are clear conflicts in some of these families regarding what we call the
level of orderliness, i.e. when the home is perceived as messy and untidy. This
could be about cleaning, how a room should look in order to pass as being tidy.
In one of the families, the woman has chosen not to take care of the cleaning.
Her husband does it, but not in the way she wishes it to be done. He does not
adapt to her norms of tidiness. It does not work out according to her wishes,
but according to him, she must accept that. Another example of a conflict of
orderliness in a family is the dishes. In this example, doing the dishes is part of
the husband's chores. The wife finds it hard to accept that plates, cutlery and
glasses pile up after dinner, and she wants her husband to do the dishes in the
evenings. He does not. It suits him better to rest at night and tackle the dishes
early in the morning. The huge pile of dishes that is left waiting for the following day does not bother him. He does deal with the dishes, but the wife thinks
he does it at the wrong time. He is not willing to change this. 'I will never do
that, it is my point of view and she has to live with that. You've got to have some
fixed norms.' In other situations, he often cedes to her wishes, but remains firm
that she must concede to him on this issue.

These examples show that men who claim to have adapted to the wishes of
their wives may claim their right to do things their way, at times. Conflicts do
still occur in these families regarding the division of labour. In some cases like
the above, it can be about the dishes, or who is to stay at home when a child is
ill or other similar issues, but fundamentally, these couples (and not in the least
the women) claim to be happy with the division of labour. However, there are
couples where the women are less satisfied, particularly those who have tried to
influence their husbands to carry more of the daily burden, but have been
unsuccessful.

Female struggle and despair

In some families, women's striving towards making the men shoulder a greater responsibility is met by resistance. The resistance expresses itself in different ways – pure inability, open unwillingness or a declared willingness to cooperate that does not translate into practice. Men can also thwart the women's ambitions by declaring a 'lower' level of orderliness. Unable to deal with this 'incompetence', the women in these families carry out the work themselves, with renewed irritation, consequent conflicts and new attempts at reaching agreements. In the power games surrounding laundry, dish washing, ironing and cleaning, a number of strategies and counter-strategies are deployed.

One of the couples formulated a division of labour at a very early stage that was adapted to the woman's work. She had actively chosen to do the shopping and the cooking, while the man did other work in the house. However, the woman claims that she is the one who is stuck with the larger part of the work, and she has periodically attempted to make her husband contribute more. These attempts to restructure the division of labour have failed. One of the battle scenes was the cleaning of the bathroom:

> And the bathroom issue, it's just that I can't take it if it's the least bit dirty. It is supposed to be clean in there. He doesn't think it's all that important if it is super-clinically clean, all the time. So he just waits, you know. He could wait for two days to clean it when it's already dirty, and I can't take it and then I do it. And the times I haven't given a crap, to see if he was going to do it, he doesn't. We have argued a whole lot about that.

Another woman has tried to make her husband do the laundry. Also this case ended up with the woman taking over the chore, because she could not handle the way her husband dealt with it:

> We have tried splitting it in other ways, but I can't take the way he handles the laundry. I don't want to send him down to the utility room. When he hangs the laundry, he just tosses it like this on the washing lines instead of pulling it. I pull the seams and hang them nicely and neatly, so that they are nice when I take them down.

During a period when her husband did the laundry, his wife really had to close her eyes when she saw how he did it:

> I could not handle it at all. I can get so irritated by the way he folds a towel. The way to fold a towel in my view is like this and like this, in three parts and then like this. He can make sausages out of them.

> *Interviewer*: Did this mean you did not let him carry on with the laundry?

Yes, at that stage, I took over. I don't want sweaters that are completely screwed up, crooked, twisted and wrinkly.

Naturally, these conflict areas can be viewed from different perspectives. One perspective is that the women's expectations of the level of quality have hindered them from achieving the desired division of labour. Another perspective is that the men seem to be unwilling to come closer to the women's demands, and have thus perhaps made use of an incompetence that has been advantageous to them. Yet another perspective is that it is the women who actively espouse the norms. The men are aware of this, but are simultaneously not willing to accept these norms. Discussions about minimal requirements that would be potentially accepted by both parties are thus not developed. In this case, both parties are able to retain 'their' control, without creating a jointly shared control. A further perspective is that since it is often the women who have the main responsibility for the household labour they end up as project managers – they make the decisions, they make the demands and they often set the requirements. Thus it becomes a question of authority. In some cases men reject or evade this authority, for various reasons – one of them perhaps being that it resembles a parental (motherly) authority. This brings us to the unconscious roles occupied by family members in the family system, and is reflective of any asymmetries that exist there.

In one case, where both partners have very long working days, it is clear that the woman carries the entire responsibility of planning, and performs most of the work in the home. The husband has certain areas of responsibility, such as shopping, but he does little else. The woman is not contented. She has long discussions with her husband about how he should contribute more, particularly in areas that concern him directly. She wants him to put things back in the right place, iron his own laundry, cook his own food when he gets back late and so on. From time to time she has outbursts about the husband contributing so little to the household work, and she knows that he gets a guilty conscience over it:

It's not like he doesn't want to help out, but . . . it's not like that most of the time. But for some reason, men don't really have the ability to carry on working when they come home! That surprises me. So we often have discussions about it, and then he tries to improve.

However, the changes are far too small, and she does not have the answer to how she can make her husband change. The gender factor is viewed as a possible explanation – that men lack the ability to work when they are home. Nagging and constant attempts at improvement have become her method, and the perspective is lifelong. 'I see this as a lifelong task to nag and then I guess things will improve.' Her view is that a certain improvement can be traced over the years, but her frustration remains great. The countless discussions do not lead to much, but the big outbursts of rage may have some effect:

Sometimes I feel like I'm nagging about certain things countless times, but the penny doesn't drop. And it's very sad that it has to get that way so that you collapse and lose your marbles completely. But sometimes it may be necessary, because it seems like that is the thing that slowly gives results anyway.

In some of the families, ironing is a source of deep frustration among the women. In one of the couples, where the man did not even iron his own work clothes, the woman discussed this issue in depth. When asked if she was the one doing his ironing, she replied:

Yes, and I don't like to hear myself say that, because I think it is *disgustingly* boring to iron. And he wears shirts to work, work shirts, you know, and they have to be ironed. And quite a lot of shirts are used. There are lots of discussions. But for some reason, it hasn't really got very far.

The practice of division of labour varies substantially in these couples. In some families, the man contributes somewhat to the household labour, but not to the extent that the woman wishes for. One couple appears in practice to have a mainly gender-based labour division that is in sharp contrast to the equal gender ideology that the woman represents. It is uncertain whether the conditions surrounding the labour division will change in the direction that the women hope for. Instead, the solution will perhaps be that they surrender and accept the existing order. Alternatively, if the men make small 'improvements', the women will interpret them as big improvements and thus become satisfied – as described in Hochschild's (1989) illustration (see Chapter 2). Conflicts can of course also be solved by the dissolution of the relationship. Discontent with the husband's efforts for jointly shared work is an important reason why women choose to divorce (Wadsby and Swedin 1993).

The description thus far may give the impression that only women direct or try to direct their men, who follow their lead with more or less reluctance. This gives a skewed picture. In reality, complex processes of cooperation and resistance (interaction and counteraction), strategies and counter-strategies are at work. Men who passively or actively, consciously or unconsciously resist taking responsibility for a greater part of the household work are in fact directing the division of labour to a large extent – including the women's frustration over the failure to create changes. None of these men claims to want a different division of labour than the one that their women want. Everybody thinks that it should be 'equal'. One of the men says that he does as much work as the woman, and has thus a different view of reality. Others say that the division of labour is unequal, and provide various explanations without defending their own behaviour pattern. Simultaneously, through their behaviour these men display that they have another model of labour division in mind than their women's.

In these relationships, battles based on gender ideology have been staged for several years. The men do not grant their women's wishes for another division of household labour, despite the fact that many of them express in words that it should be more equal. When these men and women attempt to explain this lack of justice, they often focus on some kind of inability of the man. It may be an inability fostered already in childhood, something that is related to the individual man's specific personality or men's deficiency in general. Holter and Aarseth (1994) perceive these various forms of inactivity on behalf of the men as counter-strategies to the women's attempts at creating norms in the home. Performing what women demand can be seen as subordination from the male perspective, a subordination that they resist. Given the content in the dominating gender ideology – that relationships should be equal – it is impossible for the man to confess that he actually does not want to live up to these norms. In this case, it is more acceptable to come across as a person lacking in competence, with an inability to learn. Holter and Aarseth's (1944) interpretation brings out underlying dimensions of the power games of the genders.

However, there are examples of men who give rise to a kind of equal division of labour that the female party is not prepared for.

Male independence and household labour

An example of one couple in the sample shows how both the husband and wife claim to be helping each other constantly; the man is as active in the household as the woman. They have no conflicts regarding the household labour, and they have never had any. But the woman does not take the credit for this. It is the opposite. When they moved in together, she was fully prepared to perform a great deal of household chores that she thought was expected of her, and which her mother had always done. She was surprised to see her husband take part in so many chores. Initially, she felt certain ambivalence in the matter:

> I know that I reacted to the fact that he did so much, I know that. Maybe a little surprised that he did so much. Somehow you could think – not that it was difficult – but I hadn't expected it. I thought it was given that I should do certain things. I grew up in a house where my dad never did anything. He never went shopping, he never cleaned, and he never cooked. He did the dishes occasionally. But then again he took care of a few other things. The car and the cellar and so on. So that's why I have never seen a man be so active in the home. It wasn't difficult, but a bit unusual in the beginning. I wasn't unsure of what I should be doing, but I still thought I should be doing more household chores. You get used to everything.

With these expectations and a state of alert, how come she did not take over the household work and did what her mother did? Her answer to that question was that her husband would have stopped her.

He would probably not have allowed it, because he likes doing certain things. Even the necessary evils, like cleaning and stuff like that. But he never let it go and made me do it all.

According to her own judgement, she lives in an equal relationship, but does not approve of gender debates. She states that you have to accept that the genders are different and that it has consequences. She and her husband never had such discussions. It has been 'natural' for both of them, she says, but then she changes her statement and says that it has been primarily natural for him. The background lies in his independence, according to her:

He has been very independent and was that way already when we met, so I was very surprised that he did so much.

Her husband also emphasises his wish to be independent and manage household work. This is important for him to feel as an independent person.

Doing things in the home, I don't know. It's about *being allowed* to be independent. My parents never kept the lid on, they trusted me, that I can take care of myself, manage my economy, manage hygiene, that I take care of myself, everything.

Furthermore, he says that he could never move in with a woman who would not allow him to take part in the household work. In his view, it is a matter of independence and respect:

I think it's about respect. I can actually do things around the house. I can be interested even though I'm a guy. But if I have a partner who presupposes that I cannot or will not – I would develop an ulcer within a week.

This husband associates independence with the ability to also manage household duties. He has, perhaps through his dominance, put pressure on his wife to achieve a more equal organisation of labour than she ever dreamt or asked for, not to mention fought for.[2] This situation occurs in one of the couples. In other words, it is not frequent in our limited sample, but still worthy of description as a practical possibility. There is another man with a similar position in one of the other couples. He also regards the ability to handle household chores as a sign of independence.

Associating household work with independence is probably an alien prospect to most women. However, being a good housekeeper who cleans and cooks can be a source of pride for a woman, because it confirms her competence and perhaps even femininity. But it hardly confirms her independence. On the contrary, some men have created an association between independence and household labour. Mastering household skills means that you can take care of yourself, if necessary. In that regard, independence has been achieved. When household labour is associated with the positive connotations that independence carries, the genderised circumstances of the household also change. It is not represented as women's duties, but as activities that independent people engage in. It can be regarded as an example of how associations between gender and household labour are reconstructed and given new connotations at a discourse level.

Traditionalism and female governance

In the couples presented hitherto, there is an active direction towards something we associate with 'equal' division of labour. Yet, in some couples, the women actively uphold a characteristically traditional or gender-complementary labour division.[3] Their areas of responsibility are children and the household, while the men earn money and carry out what is regarded as male duties: repairs and solving technical problems. In the framework of this order, however, the women demand a significant contribution of work carried out in the home from the men.

Both parties in these couples maintain that the women have the higher authority in family issues. The women strongly emphasise their need to have control over things in the home, the planning and whatever concerns the children. Despite this, they have made sure that their men take a relatively large responsibility for the household work as well. The couples do not have a history of disputes regarding the division of household labour.

In one of the couples, the man was used to a typical gender-based division of labour from previous relationships, and had been 'waited on like a king'. In the current relationship, he had to get used to doing a whole lot more. Both spouses even claim that he does more than the wife. He cleans, helps the children with their homework and other things, and repairs the house and his parents' house. Weekends and evenings when the wife is at work, he takes care of the household and the children, cooks, does the dishes, keeps things tidy and makes sure that the children get to bed. When the wife is at home, she does all of these tasks. The home is not his but her responsibility. It appears that the spouses have different ways of running the household, the children and their bedtime. When the wife is at home, her principles dictate how the household is run.

To summarise, the household and the children are the wife's responsibility when she is at home. The husband's work is to repair and renovate the house. He thinks that she could contribute to the comprehensive renovation works that are entirely up to him. His wish that she would work with him is not only about speeding up the renovation. It would also be more fun to work together:

> She could definitely help so that it gets underway a bit . . . And somebody who had taken part and helped more. It would be more fun, too.

In other words, he would like a more collaborative partnership. But she is not interested. She is the one who actively upholds the division of labour in strictly female and male spheres. The men are allowed into the female sphere when necessary, though.

In another couple, the woman principally carries out all household work, although the husband took care of the children when the wife was in paid work. The woman has always made all plans, keeping tabs of everything, including the finances. Her husband confirms this, and says that their division of labour is very 'uneven'. 'My wife does more or less everything. I try to keep up.' But his wife is content and would not want it any other way. She works fewer hours and thinks that it is reasonable that she puts more into the household labour. That is not her only reason, though. It is as important to her that she has the main responsibility for the work in the house. 'If someone were to take it from me I would feel terrible.' Exactly what is so terrible to lose?

> The control, I think. I would like to have control over things. Not in an exaggerated way, absolutely not, but I want to know how things are and that's that.

To this woman, the important thing is to know that her husband can take care of duties in the home if she is travelling, for instance. If she wants to, he can take over. Two things emerge as particularly important to her. The first is to uphold the image of herself in the centre of the home. The second is that the man and the children should not take it for granted that she does everything, even if she actually does. In her own words, 'I don't have a stamp on my forehead that says that these are my chores!' These two things are important elements in her perceptive construction of them as an equal couple. On his side, the husband helps her maintain this image. He often expresses his gratitude over how much she takes care of. In perhaps a somewhat apologetic tone, he says to the interviewer that he would like to do more. But he always lags behind in his attempts compared to the wife, who is so much faster and more effective in all her undertakings in their home.

These are examples of women who actively maintain a model of labour division that appears as very gender traditional, but at the same time they make sure that the men make efforts in the home, sometimes in significant proportions. This model is not easily slotted into the current discussions of equality. The potential source of conflict in couples that apply a traditional framework of gender-complementarity in the division of labour is that the women make sure that the men carry out some of the female duties.

Thus far, we have seen examples of women who more or less successfully have attempted to direct their husbands towards a more equal work model. We have also seen one man gearing towards a more equal labour division, and finally an active female governance towards a gender-traditional labour division. Next, we shall describe examples of a more jointly shared value basis of men and women in terms of issues of household division of labour.

Both parties govern

The mutual collaborators

We refer to one group of couples as the 'mutual collaborators'. When it comes to household work in this case, both parties present a picture of collaboration, satisfaction and an actual absence of conflicts surrounding the issue. None of them have campaigned for the existing order, which instead seems to have emerged by itself, sometimes even from the very start.

In one couple, the wife works part time and the husband works irregular shifts. When he is off work, it is a matter of course that he deals with the laundry and ironing, and during cleaning sessions, he wipes the tables and windowpanes, as well as removing any stains on the doors. The tasks follow a flow that lacks strict divisions of male and female lines of duty, although one party performs one type of task more often than the other.

Another couple provides an example where the husband has a history of contributing less, but has gradually increased his efforts. His wife has neither fought nor resisted it.

> I don't take it for granted that he should do the things he does, but he still does them. That is the way it should work – helping each other – without nagging.

The husband in another couple places particular emphasis on how they work as a 'team'. The implication is that the work in the home is not split in an exact way: 'What needs to be done is done.' Each person contributes when necessary. The woman in this case claims that she instigates the work, but on the whole, they come through for each other. From the stories told by these men and women, it is evident that men perform a significant part in the household work, although the women are said to do more or have the 'superior responsibility'.

The question is then: have the women just been lucky when choosing their partner? Or do they contribute in any way? What would have happened if the men had not been active? In that case, would the women have tried to direct them?

Starting with the last question, we suspect that there is no unambiguous answer. The woman who claims not to expect very much of the man would perhaps not have tried to reshape his behaviour. The other two women present a different picture, however. Both of them make it very clear that they would never have accepted a man who does not live up to 'his' share of the household labour. One of them refers to her father as the role model. Her mother worked full time and the father often cooked and cleaned. Being used to such men, she expected nothing less in her own relationship. The other woman came from a previous marriage where both she and her husband had entered traditional gender roles from the very start. She had been 'pottering around' like most women do. The division of labour was fixed from the beginning, and was later impossible to change. After a couple of years, she broke from this pattern that she was absolutely determined not to repeat it in her new relationship – and she did not, either. Yet, we do not know what the women would have done if their men had not lived up to their expectations. According to them, they never had to fight for an equal division of labour. It emerged by itself.

On the basis of our material, we do not get closer to the answer of this question of equality. It is possible to extract themes and contemplate their relevance only in the circumstances provided. One such relevance is the importance of having a similar view of the good 'orderliness' of the household. Several men in these couples maintain that they are rather pedantic. They think orderliness is important, and in some cases the women claim that the men are tidier than they are. It is an open question whether this is of any relevance. One of the men in this group associates his involvement in household labour with independence.

Another theme is constituted by women's thoughts about themselves in relation to having a family. 'Us women', one of them says, 'are phenomenal in getting caught up on the small things'. She becomes irritated when her husband leaves the newspaper in the bathroom or puts the cheese in the breadbox. She perceives displaying irritation over such things as a typical female trait, something which she rejects. Discerning between the petty and the important is the real issue at stake. Another woman says that she perceives her whole life as a series of negotiations and compromises. She describes herself as a good compromiser:

> We can compromise and balance things. I am not full of prestige so that I say 'No way, I have to!' But sure, I can be grumpy.

She started her family late in life and has given up many previous ambitions. In her view, that is part of the price for good togetherness in a family, a 'luxury' that is worth many a compromise.

Generosity is another emphasised theme. One woman does not like strict divisions and always having to ask who does what:

> You have to give a little. And it doesn't have to be that important who does what, I don't think so. The main thing is that both see what has to be done.'

The 'giving' theme is also emphasised by another woman. In a relationship, you do not give and take: 'Both should give, and that makes it better.' She exemplifies this with an everyday-type event. On one occasion, when she was coming home after work, she was looking forward to eating a potato salad that she had kept in the fridge. When she called home, she was told it was finished, and that the husband and children had eaten it. When she arrived home, her husband had gone out and bought her a new salad. With this example, she wanted to illustrate the care, giving and generosity in relation to one another in everyday life.

A possible explanation for men's greater activity could be that the women in these couples create norms to a lesser extent than the governing but frustrated women. Could it be that the women do not challenge a male sensitivity to being governed and therefore also provide more space for the men's terms? These questions have to remain open, since no definite answers can be provided from this study.

The traditional

Some of the couples where both parties direct have a division of labour that is clearly gender-complementary. It took shape as the relationship was initiated: 'It just ended up that way', as many of them express it. What these couples have in common is that the woman has the main responsibility for the household labour, and executes the majority of the chores. The man assists to some extent, often performing certain tasks that have become his. A clear division of 'female' and 'male' reigns here, female and male spheres of labour exist of which the respective gender influences the circumstances. The women have shouldered the greater part of the work in the home, and perceive it as inevitable. Some claim to be content with their situation; others express irritation or desperate discontent.

From the very start in these couple relationships, there has been a mutually shared view of the division of labour that splits the traditionally female duties from the male, each gender performing accordingly. This has occurred despite the fact that the women in some of the cases work full time. With time, this division of labour has aroused their irritation, but the pattern seems to be difficult to change. The social situations in these families are so different that it is possible to discern variations. In one of the families, a parent of one of the partners participates in the household work, which obviously creates special circumstances. Families in which both parties work full time operate under different circumstances than families in which the woman works part time.

Both parties work full time

In some couples, both the husband and the wife work full time. The woman takes on the main part of the household labour. She cooks, does the dishes, cleans, tidies, helps the children with their homework, buys their clothes and sometimes also shops for groceries.

Even though the division of labour is gender-complementary according to a traditional pattern, there are some cases where women perform duties that are associated with the male sphere. They repair broken items, install and attach items to the walls, etc. One woman refuses to leave similar things to her husband, solely because 'it is men's work, I won't do it. Anything that he can fix, I can do it as well.' Another woman carries out all redecoration work inside the house, such as putting up wallpaper or painting. All of these couples live in one-family houses with a garden attached. The gardening is either the complete responsibility of the woman, or in some cases shared with the man. In other words, additionally to the traditional female work, the women also perform 'men's work'. As one woman puts it:

> If you want to divide the chores into male and female, I think I do the female and he does the male. Being really mean about it, I think I do more male than he does female. That is if you consider gardening to be male, but it is pretty heavy duty.

So what do the men do? They drive the children to their leisure activities – hockey, football, table tennis and dance – and sometimes stay to watch. Some men are heavily engaged in the children's activities, for example attending matches (but so do the women). Men also sometimes help the children with their homework. If large items in the household break, the men deal with it. It could be the oil tank or the front outdoor staircase breaking down, a room that has to be renovated or a bathroom that has to be renewed. The entire house may be gradually renovated over the course of many years, and the car has to be maintained. Acquiring technical equipment is a predominantly male task. Over the course of several years, one husband had nagged his wife about buying a dishwasher, which she resisted at length. Another man took the initiative to install a central vacuum cleaner. Purchasing television sets and stereos is also typically male. But this is not specific to these families; it also applies to the other families.

These men also transcend into the sphere of traditionally female duties. Several men do the weekly shopping or (sometimes) cook at the weekends. When the children were in day-care, they also picked up or dropped off the children occasionally. Very occasionally, some men also vacuum clean – which caused a child to burst out in surprise: 'But daddy, are you cleaning?!' One of the men emphasises that he actually irons his own shirts. His wife refuses to do it for him, saying that despite the fact that she does so much around the house, he should really do that himself!

What are the reasons given for this traditional division of labour? Let us begin with the men's motives for not participating in the female sphere. Both self-criticism and apologies can be discerned in their arguments.

One reason presented is that the woman demands too much. She is excessively cleanliness-conscious and will not tolerate 'dust bunnies', whereas the man is not bothered by 'a bit of crap here and there.' The woman has a greater need for a clean house, and initiates the cleaning on her own accord. Another reason presented is that the wife has more drive and is more of a matron/housekeeper. It is never expressed directly, but the implication is that many of the things that the wife does are through her own choice and the husband does not consider them to be necessary. The underlying message is that she has herself to blame. However, the husband presents himself as more pressured by work and their economy than the wife, sometimes working weekends and evenings. Other reasons relate to a lack of household demands from the family of origin. One man carries the image of his father who always left the table without removing anything, and never contributed. Yet another reason is lack of competence. For example, he does not know how to wash clothes, because he never had the experience.

To summarise, we have here an entire selection of reasons that point to the fact that the skewed division of labour is something that the husband cannot really be blamed for. On the other hand, there are also instances of self-criticism in the men's reasoning. Their reasons don't even appear plausible to themselves. One husband, who refers to the pressures of his work, adds: 'It could be that you hide behind your work, and say that you are too tired or don't have time.' 'Work' is used to shirk from the second shift at home. One man claims that he has put off doing chores that have been agreed with the wife, that it 'perhaps was comfortable' since the wife in those cases took over the chore.

What about the women – how do they think? Their reasoning includes not only duty and freedom, control and exclusion, but also self-reproach. They differ from the men in how they accept their situation.

One woman takes care of the laundry, because 'then it is done my way, the way I want it.' It is the same case with the cleaning: 'He cleans in a way that I don't accept, so I do it instead.' She has not wanted to 'let him in' on certain duties, such as doing the laundry and cleaning. She appears to think that the full responsibility for the laundry gives her control. She can decide when it is done and when she lets it accumulate into large piles. At times, she becomes very irritated and feels overworked, but she is determined to maintain the order that she wants.

Another woman is no longer pleased with the division of labour in the house, but is unable to see how it could change. Somebody has to do the things that have to be done, such as cleaning and laundry. Since the husband does not care if the house is messy, it becomes her duty:

> I haven't really had a choice, because he doesn't give a crap. Somebody has to do it and so I have sacrificed other things because you can't do everything.

The sense of duty for what has to be done is strongly emphasised here. The irritation she carries seldom causes open conflicts, because in her experience, they do not lead anywhere.

Another woman is deeply discontented with her situation. She argues back and forth about how she has tried to change the situation, but essentially, these are strategies of how she is trying to change herself. She has to learn how to speak her mind and argue, and not become upset and cry. But she has also considered other strategies, such as refraining from performing certain responsibilities that have become exclusively hers:

I have two full-time jobs. I could let go of some things. I could let the laundry just sit there, and finally they won't have any clean underwear.

But she adds that she is not like that:

If I'm going to wash my panties then I might as well throw in his underwear, that's the way it is.

The fantasy about a family revolution is stopped short by practical everyday chores.

When asked if they have conflicts about the division of labour, she replies:

No, conflicts [long pause]. I guess I have more or less accepted things, and nothing can be done about it. I've come so far that [sigh] I don't give a crap. I let it be messy. I don't make demands on myself, either, because I don't think my husband can make demands on having an orderly house since he doesn't do anything about it either. It's my way of solving it – I also let it go.

She has no faith in changing him, and so she changes herself. She cares less about the household. Since he doesn't do anything either, she can stop keeping things tidy. She is lessening the demands on herself.

An important distinction between her and the frustrated women who try to direct their men towards greater participation is that she is fundamentally placing the blame on herself. 'I'm a bit bad at delegating, so it's a lot to do with me.' 'It's partly my fault, I am aware of that.' The guilt is also part of the other two women's thinking. If the man does not see the need for clean laundry, then the woman has to take it on. And then it becomes partly her guilt: 'It is my fault, I've let things slide.' If she was not willing to let her husband in on certain chores, then she is the one to blame:

And so I can't whine, even if I do sometimes and think I have way too much to do. But at the same time, I realise that I have myself to blame. I don't confess to it all the time, but sitting like this I can.

As we have seen, the men imply that the women have themselves to blame since they make such demands on the household labour. To a certain extent, some women meet their men halfway in this type of accusation. The women also agree with their men that they have been brought up to be served and that they have become rather spoilt 'since mother did it all.' Some women say that they have replaced their men's mothers.

He has never learnt to take responsibilities and then I came in straight after the mum and took everything on myself, as well. I am aware of that.

Half-time housewives – by choice or by force

In the couples that feature a predominantly traditional division of labour, the women work half time. Most of the household work and childcare is the wife's responsibility, although the husband 'helps out' when he comes home. He sits down with the children's homework, cleans occasionally and is responsible for renovations. This is an example of a woman who feels suffocated by all the duties of the household and all its 'musts'. As opposed to the women who actively direct towards a traditional division, this woman does not appear to have made a positive choice. She works part time, but not in order to enjoy the main responsibility for children and the home. Her 'free' choice is more negative, in the sense that she has chosen not to work full time, because in her view it would be even worse:

> I haven't chosen this because I am very keen on being in this situation, but I feel better if I can take care of the children than working full time and come home and throw food into the children's mouths. I would feel terrible doing that. I think it would be very taxing to have it like that. I would rather carry this load. I anyway think I feel better than working all day and come home and be tired and exhausted.

As opposed to the women mentioned previously, this choice is not connected to the sense of being in control over the home sphere. Nor is it the case that she strives for control. Instead, she expresses a feeling of lack of control in relation to her situation. However, she has still made her choice based on the more or less explicit expectations of her as a woman to perform the larger share of the housework. This order has not been the subject of any discussions or questioning.

Two women in a household

One special couple formation is a family in which two women carry the load of the women's work, the wife and her retired mother-in-law. The paternal grandmother of the children comes to see them almost every day, helps them plan and cook meals, irons the laundry and is at home when the children come home from school. They have dinner together almost every day. In this family, the division of labour is relatively gender traditional, even though the husband shops for food, takes the children to various activities and helps out with the food and laundry on the weekends. Because of the mother-in-law's contributions, the full-time working mother gets a chance to relax a little in the evenings. She repeatedly says that it would not have been possible without her mother-in-law.

> And there is nothing [in the work at home] that I have experienced that tough and that's very much due to my mother-in-law. Because if I had had

all the other stuff, then I would not have been able to do it. But it's just because I don't have to do the ironing when I come home like many other women, since my mother-in-law would already have ironed. Things like that make me able to relax and maybe watch some TV when the kids are in bed.

This quote shows that she thinks it is natural that she, as a wife and mother, should have the responsibility for most things in the household. If the mother-in-law hadn't been there, most of the chores would have been hers to complete.

This family exemplifies what Louise Gaunt (1987) found to be rather common in a local Swedish community that she studied in the beginning of the 1980s. Relatives, mainly mothers and married daughters, were in very close contact with each other, and the mothers could help their adult children several times a week. The study shows that the older generation can be an important resource in modern families, even if they do not share households (Gaunt 1987). Borchgrevink (1995) discusses how in this case the women themselves contribute to perpetuate the conceptions of what is male and female. Borchgrevink illuminates this argument with an example from a family in which the wife did not accept all the chores expected of a woman. She demanded that the husband should carry out some of them. When she returned home after a journey, she found that the husband had not had to do anything in her absence. His mother had come to the house and performed all the female duties. The attempts to open up the home sphere and redefine the female had failed. The older woman had entered and shut it.

In the family in our sample, the older woman is a positive resource for all persons involved. Most probably, being needed is what she receives in return for her favours. The paradox – which cannot be ignored – is that she simultaneously contributes to upholding a gender-polarised division of labour.

Summarising comments

The presentation of various couples in this chapter is naturally not exhaustive. It is possible to imagine more variations than our material gives evidence of. The diffuse boundaries between the categories render the classifications arbitrary to a certain extent. For example, we can question whether the woman with a traditional division of labour described as 'desperately discontented' may not rather be an example of a despairing/impotent woman who is trying to direct the division of labour towards a greater equality. Instead, we have emphasised that she has upheld a traditional division of labour with her husband. Yet, at the time of the interview, she had begun questioning this long-established order. It is a matter not only of classification, but also of the point in time of the person's life history that one chooses to use as a basis of interpretation. The woman in this case was in transition between perspectives of her life situation, with the will to change her circumstances to better suit new needs.

We found no examples of men who openly and explicitly tried to direct the division of labour towards a more traditional order against the woman's will. These examples are indirect in the cases where the men resist the women's attempts to make them contribute more to the household labour. Yet none of them purposefully expresses such an ambition; it appears indirectly through actions. Men with a traditional division of labour do not express such wishes either. It can be compared with the women's more actively formulated ambitions to attain an equal division of labour.

The basis of this presentation is what women and men claim to be striving towards, and how they achieve their goals, in other words their ideals and practice, influence and conflicts. There are examples of couples where the women, and the men to some extent, have an explicit equal orientation, at the same time as their practice is formulated in a very gender-traditional way. The flip side of this is exemplified by couples with explicitly traditional ideals, where the man carries out a great deal of the household work in practice. In some couples, ideals and practice seem to concur. This is the case with couples who have either traditional or equal ideals. In couples where at least one party experiences a pronounced discrepancy between ideals and practice, we have observed higher levels of conflict.

The arguments we have put forward in this chapter have featured concepts such as directing and influence. We see pictures of women who try to direct their more or less resisting men to participate more in the household labour, and of women who actively choose a traditional division of labour. Such pictures give focus to the suppositions of women's liability to subordination to men. In other words, there is reason to conduct a detailed discussion on issues of influence and superior–subordinate orders in the couples that are part of this study.

Female governing and subordination

There is substantial evidence that women who see themselves as living in equal relationships put more effort into the home compared to their husbands. This is the case both for women who have fought to achieve equality in the division of labour, and women who are mutual collaborators. This means that even among couples where both claim to have a fair, balanced division of labour, the woman does the greater share of the work. Both the women's and the men's descriptions support this conclusion. The woman is often thought to have the main responsibility of the household: she is the one who does the strategic planning. In addition, almost half of the women we interviewed worked part time, and none of the men worked part time. The women who work part time do so as 60–90 per cent of a full working week. Women part-timers are included among those who have struggled to achieve an equal distribution of labour, among those who despair in their attempts to make the men take on a greater responsibility in the household, among those who have a mutually collaborative pattern and among those who have a traditional division of labour. Why have these women chosen to work part time, and what consequences does this have for the division of labour? Have they made conscious choices or been forced to choose? How can we understand the aspect of influence based on the fact that women in all categories do more of the labour in the household?

Starting with the choice to work part time – what do the women say about their choices? Only two out of ten say it has not been voluntary.[4] Other women present part-time work as something positive, as a choice they made actively. Let us look more closely at a few examples from different social classes.

One highly educated woman with a high-status job has made the choice to work part time. Ever since the children were born, she has worked 80 per cent, and claims to have made the choice

> so that I will have time to do anything at all. I always say that it's about quality of life. When I see envious looks on Thursday afternoons as I say 'Have a nice weekend' . . . well, then I say that I have a little less in salary, but it's worth it. It really feels that way.

The reduced work hours have no substantial consequences for the family economy, because the husband has a high-paying job. The woman has chosen part time because she likes it, despite the fact that she also enjoys her work and finds it stimulating:

> I want to do it. In the beginning, when I was going back to work, I was considering half time, because I really enjoyed being at home. I didn't think it was boring. I enjoyed it. But I didn't dare do it, because of the risk of not being able to work more hours later. I mean 80 per cent; I feel that we can manage living off that. I have no intention of working more in the next ten years. This suits me perfectly, and as long as we can afford it, I will do it, even when the kids get older. Because I think that both they and I need it anyway. And the family. Because of course, I can do things that are useful to the whole family when I'm free.

There are several components in this woman's comments. The first is that she works part time in order to have the time to do all the things related to the family and its needs. The second is that she views the possibility to work part time as a great privilege. It represents quality of life to her. The third (which is not apparent in this particular quote) is that she tries not to perform her household duties on her day off, despite the fact that she often ends up doing them anyway.

Another woman has a low level of education, her work is low status, but she enjoys being at work. Both she and her husband have low incomes, which renders her income indispensable to the family finances. In this family, the spouses have wanted to sort out the childcare privately, and by juggling their jobs, the children have almost never been to nursery.[5] The woman's work 'makes almost no difference'. She leaves early and gets home early. According to her, it is good to be able to cook and do the laundry during the day, and not having to do it in the evening. She thinks it is rather 'luxurious these days' and feels 'panic' at the thought of working full time and only have the evening to do housework. She has not chosen to work part time because she is 'comfortable', but because of the children.

> I always knew that this time is very short, so I feel like I want to. Time goes so fast, you know, I can work full time all my life, but these years right now, they are so important.

Part-time work gives her a smaller pay cheque, but 'I still feel like I made this choice for my own sake, for the children and for the family. If I felt like I wanted to work more, I would probably have made an effort towards it.'

Part-time work is viewed by this woman as her own choice, something she has done for the children and the family. She experiences luxury with it in her everyday life, and does not look forward to working full time.

Do these women really have the influence over their situation to the extent that they express? A central question in this case is if the choice to work part time is based on their premises and goals, or if it is based on subordination to the needs of the family and the husband. Do these women in reality adapt to the needs of others and are they subordinate to their men?

According to the theoretical perspectives represented by Haavind (1982), Cheal (1991), Holmberg (1993), Bourdieu (1999), among others, male dominance is central in all relationships between men and women. This is true of couple relationships and families. Compared to earlier epochs, the male domination is no longer as visible and manifest, but more implicit. This is also the case in couple relationships. With equality as the dominating ideology, male power can no longer be exerted openly. In this more veiled shape, it becomes unclear also to the involved parties and is not identified as exertion of power. This means that what may seem as a free choice or wish to the woman could be a form of self-deception. She does not see that, in reality, she is adapting her actions according to the needs of the man, and thereby subordinating to him. The relationship orientation of women, seeing to the needs of others and what is good for the relationship, contributes to strengthen the tendency to subordination. This perspective thus gives reason to doubt the women's descriptions when they claim that it was their choice to work part time and do more of the housework.

An alternative perspective claims that the women do not always adapt their actions and decisions according to the needs of the children and the husbands. Women can have their own goals that they want to realise within the family sphere, and in some cases the man must be subordinate. Thagaard (1996) claims that in the understanding of female influence in families, we must take into account women's possibility of choice, their motivation, what they want and wish for. There is a great difference between taking care of the house and the children, although you do not really want to, and being at home if you feel like it. Thagaard (1996) and also Bjerrum Nielsen and Rudberg (1994) emphasise the difference between want and necessity, and view it as determining what women want and what they can realise. There are a number of factors that limit or expand a woman's possibility of choice when it comes to full-time or part-time work. Levels of income, interesting work possibilities and access to good childcare are all factors that lie outside the family. In the family, however, the man is an important factor. If he performs household labour unwillingly, or puts a premium on his own career, then he limits the woman's possibility of choice. If, on the other hand, the man is willing to do a substantial part of the housework, the woman is granted a possibility to act. If she still chooses to work part time instead of full time, it is doubtful whether she is subordinated to the husband. It could be the case that she acts according to her own preferences.

Thagaard (1996), similarly to Holter and Aarseth (1994), claims that many women more or less consciously wish to be in the centre of the family. By performing the larger part of the work and taking a greater responsibility, a woman can create and uphold a central position, whereas the man occupies a more peripheral position. Sharing the central position with the man can be associated with feelings of ambivalence in the woman. Women's extra work in the home, where the needs of others are given priority in relation to their own needs, can be a strategy to create and uphold a central position. Women's relationship-oriented work can be a means to gain influence and control within the family. The tendency of women to do more work in the home, and consider the needs of others before their own, can be interpreted in two diametrically opposing ways. From one perspective, this behaviour orientation can be seen as women's subordination to the man, the children and their needs. Women give more than they get in return, which denotes a relationship of exploitation (see for example Jónasdóttir 1991). From another perspective, it has another implication. The same actions can be seen as women's strategies to increase their influence in the family, to create their own central position. Giving more than you receive is a way of creating power. It can also be compared to what characterises good leadership in an organisation. The good leader tries to take everybody's interests into account and is responsible to ensure that the totality is functioning (Thagaard 1996: 29–39; see also Holter and Arseth 1994).

Returning to our previous examples, it is our opinion that the choice made by these women to work part time does not unequivocally imply that they are subordinated to their men. They actually have alternative routes of action. One of the women has an interesting job, her children are in after-school care, and the man does a lot of the household work. She does more than he does, but she also says that she wants to have the main responsibility for everybody in the family, including her husband. Another woman is hardly subordinated to the needs of the man, but rather to what she perceives to be the needs of the children. This woman occupies a strong central position in the home and expresses very clearly her wish to be in control over the home and the children. However, there are cases in our material where the women seem to have made the choice to work part time in a situation that is almost forced. In these cases, the lack of help from the man has limited her possibilities of choice, along with perceptions of household work as female duties. Here it is reasonable to claim that the woman is subordinated to the man and to perpetuated gender norms. Full-time working women, who due to duty and 'sour necessity' serve their husbands in terms of different types of care work, also give in to a certain type of subordination.

Another factor where gender determines the range of choice is that women find it less problematic to choose part-time work, something which men do not. This has nothing to do with specific couple relationships, but is connected to the gender ideologies that exist on all levels of society. These ideologies, or normative structures, are naturally very important because they affect salary levels and labour markets, as well as women's and men's wishes and needs. They limit both men's and women's possibilities to act, but in different ways. Men who would like to work part time in order to spend more time with the children and the home probably have to overcome greater obstacles in order to realise it. These obstacles lie within themselves, in the couple relationship and in society as a whole.

An overarching conclusion of this discussion is that there is no generally applicable pattern of interpretation that accounts for women's part-time work or their extra household work. In any case, we cannot accept that *one* explanation of superiority and subordination is relevant in all cases. Neither can we assume that it is a case of purposeful achievement of goals. It has not been our aim to explain the patterns of division of labour presented in this chapter. The aim has been to highlight the actual variation in patterns. The purpose was thus restricted to describing different types of ideals and practices, different ways of handling issues that concern an equal division of labour in the household. In Chapter 6, we will shed light on the construction of equality in more detail.

Chapter 6

How is equality in division of labour created?

We divided the work very clearly at an early stage, so we don't need to get irritated. If you have decided upon areas of responsibility, then I think you have to accept the way he cleans, I think so.

We kind of divide it, like the cleaning. He vacuums a lot then, he tidies up a lot more than I do.

My personal view is that it is such a drag to distinguish what is mine and what is yours. I think it depends on how things are, what goes on that day. You should share it, but I'm a little against things like 'vacuuming is actually your job.'

We have never had any conflicts about who does what, but things work out naturally.

No, it's not like we have sat down and made a division. It ended up this way. I like living so that things end up [a certain way]. Because they do anyway.

It just ended up this way.

The quotes above exemplify three ways of talking about division of labour and equality. The first way emphasises that equality is reached by splitting the work and agreeing upon who does what. Women and men who espouse this say that they have come to good solutions of real or potential conflicts through such agreements. Agreements regarding the division of labour in the household are viewed as something good and desirable, as important aspects of an equal relationship. The subsequent quotes emphasise the 'spontaneous' or 'natural' ways of the process of dividing the work. No agreements are necessary to split the chores, it should work itself out. In both these ways of speaking, there is a normative dimension about how a good division of labour should look and be created. The final quotes are not as normative. Division of labour is described as something which ended up that way. 'It just ended up this way' is a common way of making statements about the emergence of the division of labour. It seems to have taken its own shape and has not been the object of reflection. It is often a way to express that the work order is gender-traditional in its organisation, and is shaped according to conventional expectations.

It is our view that these ways of talking about division of labour reflect different equality ideals. Those that put a premium to agreements value negotiation, entering a contract about ways of addressing the daily chores. We refer to this as a contract-oriented ideal of addressing division of labour. Those whose view it is that the division of labour should solve itself, emphasise the spontaneous elements, the mutuality of the togetherness and that each person should see to common needs. We call this the needs-oriented division of labour. The third approach – 'It just ended up this way' – is in practice associated with a gender-determined division of labour. There is an implicit or rarely openly expressed morality dictating that women and men should carry out different chores according to their gender.

The various approaches to the creation of the division of labour in the home are made concrete later in this chapter. We will have a closer look at what is meant by an equal division of labour, and what it may entail. What do people take into account when they try to ascertain whether their division of labour is fair or unfair? What principles are used when reaching the conclusion? As we will see, not just one principle is used, but several sometimes conflicting principles are used.

In the following section, we will look more deeply into the issue of these principles. Our analysis is based on the interviewees' descriptions of how and why they have divided the household labour in particular ways, and their reflections about the determinants of fairness and unfairness. From ways of speaking about household work, reflections and rationales regarding division of labour, ideals, norms and rules frequently emerge indirectly. Five principles can be discerned that are used both in perception of justice and in rationales for creating a particular type of labour division. These are doing equal amounts (i.e. sameness in work efforts); displaying a jointly shared responsibility; dividing up labour according to the pleasure principle (what you like and do not like); being competent (what you can and cannot do); acknowledging a traditional gender division of labour (what are regarded as specifically male and female tasks).

Principles of justice behind divisions of labour

Doing equal amounts: the issue of measurement

In Chapter 2, we claimed that the public discussion of equality has been carried out in terms of sameness – in other words, 'how many' and 'how much'. The notion of sameness is also an important aspect of the concepts of fairness/justice, that justice is achieved when everybody in a group is treated the same, is given equal amounts or must make the same efforts. Although it is not the only implication of justice, it is a central part of the equality ideal.

In considering whether the division of labour in the household is equal, some men and women emphasise the aspect of sameness. Each person should have similar duties for equality to be achieved, or must put in the same effort in terms of time. For example: one woman thinks that she and her husband have an equal division of labour, because they perform roughly the same amounts of household chores. Another woman has the opinion that both parties should spend as much time doing household chores. However, it is not regarded as important that you do the same things, because it is sameness in time, not in task, that is counted. Several interviewees maintain that the work efforts may vary over time, but equal out in the long-term perspective. 'You put in efforts over time, but things even out in the long run' is something that both men and women claim. In these different ways of referring to equality, the importance of each person's contribution, at least in the long-term perspective, is consistently emphasised. The principle of sameness is highlighted.

Strikingly, there are many reservations in regards to applying principles of sameness. Many claim that it is unreasonable to do exactly the same things. Many also reject the actual thinking behind it. 'I do not like thinking in terms of complementing or compensating,' one woman said. Keeping track of the pluses and minuses does not constitute the determining factor; the quality and the fact that both contribute does, as one woman puts it. Some protest against what they refer to as 'millimetre fairness'. 'Performing exactly the same and being exactly fair is not important.' Women in particular have reservations about different types of divisions: 'Dividing so that you take that part and you take the other is no good.' Or: 'If fairness is that both do the same things as much, then fairness is not important.' 'Measuring with a ruler' is disliked. Women and men who either have a gender-traditional division of labour or what we refer to as mutual collaboration are the ones with reservations and direct rejections of the sameness notion.

Performing exactly equal amounts of household chores is thus regarded by some as an unacceptable principle of division. Some openly resist applying a principle of justice that implies weighing and measuring, and offsetting the efforts against each other. Two rationales for these reservations are provided. One takes into account the difficulty in comparing different efforts, and is thus attributed to a rational basis. The other has a moral ground, and states that the notion itself is inconvenient.

The first qualification can be exemplified by a man who claims to have difficulties determining whether the division of labour is fair, because he does not know what is counted as household labour. Should he include the actual 'physical labour', or should he also include the woman's planning and preparedness, which he does not contribute to? Or as one woman put it: 'How do you compare cleaning with taking the kids to the football practice?' Should you count the length in time, or also take into account that certain things may be more pleasurable? And how do these factors outweigh each other? Other couples also express the difficulty of judging how much each person contributes in terms of jointly shared duties. These difficulties are given a rational basis. They are presented as if it was a matter of performing a calculation, which is not possible in practice.

The other qualification has nothing to do with difficulties of calculation, but is related to morals. Here, it is claimed that the sameness principle goes against a moral norm stating that in couple relationships, you should not weigh and measure efforts to offset them against each other. This is associated with feelings of envy, monitoring and control. One woman points out that she measures her own or her husband's efforts in the home only when she is irritated and cranky. She openly admits that it is 'a sad way of thinking about it' and dislikes the fact that she sometimes applies it. It is as if the implication is a violation of the founding principles in a love relationship.

The statements about dividing the household labour equally is thus characterised by a great deal of ambivalence. Emphasis is placed on the principle of equal division on the one hand, and on the norm against calculating and measuring the contributions made to the jointly shared on the other.

This is an expression of what Kaufmann (1992) refers to as the gift economy in couple relationships (see Chapter 3). Calculating and accounting are opposed to the idea of a primary and fundamental togetherness, and being part of a close relationship. Thoughts on performing the same amount of work, measured in time or task, are still prevalent in several couples in some shape or form. Yet, reservations and hesitations prevail. It is as if there were two types of justice thinking, where one accepts the notion of sameness and the other does not.

When efforts are weighed against each other – in open discussions or quietly to oneself – it could imply the onset of questioning the relationship, a process that could lead to separation. This argument is led by Barbro Lennéer-Axelson, who quotes the following poem by Maria Wine in her discussions of different types of negotiation strategies. The poem expresses distrust of the notion of sameness in regards to love relationships:

> Do not question which one of you gave more
> Or pulled the hardest
> The scale is the enemy of love –
> If you require its balance, it is no longer a matter of love.[1]

Displaying a jointly shared responsibility

An important point of departure in judging whether a relationship is equal is the question if both take a jointly shared responsibility for the family and the household. The display of both parties' mutuality is mentioned by almost all male and female interviewees as being important. What does this mutuality mean in practice?

The principle is expressed in different ways. According to two men, the responsibility of everything in the home must be shared by both parties. 'We share everything,' another man says, 'it is immoral not to share.' 'Each of us takes part in the daily work.' An important aspect of the jointly shared responsibility is also said to include looking after each others' needs: 'It is important to make sure that each of us gets what they need and nobody feels like they are lacking something.' The implication is that if both man and woman are attentive to what needs to be done – and make sure it is done – a mutual responsibility is displayed. Taking full responsibility does not mean that you do the same things, nor does it mean that you perform as much in terms of time or task. The sameness principle is not at all emphasised. The following quote expresses this: 'I do not like dividing; instead there should be a spirit of helping and shared responsibility.' A jointly shared responsibility is presented as absolutely fundamental. Frustration will arise if one party experiences a deficiency in the other in this regard.

One woman in a couple who employ a traditional division of labour is particularly ambivalent in her statements about her and her husband's efforts for the common good. According to her, there is an imbalance between them in this regard. This becomes particularly obvious to her when she cleans and tidies while he does nothing. The situation puts pressure on her and she prefers the man to stay away:

> I think it is stressful to see him walking around with his hands in his pockets when I am toiling away. It is more like that. I think we have a pretty good male–female division in the home and I don't think it's wrong, as long as both do something. It shouldn't be that one lies on the sofa and the other one is working to death.

The same theme is mentioned by other women. Both have to make an effort for the common good, so that one person does not end up with all the work and the other one relaxes. One of the women, who after many years' struggle has achieved an equal division of labour, claims that they do not accept a situation where only one person is toiling. She does not like measuring with a ruler so that everything is fair and just. In her view, the issue is that 'both should take responsibility to do what is needed.' This view includes looking after not only your own, but also the needs of the other. Since the needs may change over time, the orientation should be flexible. If one party needs extra help in the household work, the other should be able to recognise this and contribute.

Displaying jointly shared responsibility may in practice mean that both parties engage in activities of different kinds, but are regarded by both as beneficial to the togetherness. One partner may for instance drive the children to their leisure activities, while the other one cleans. One of them may be doing paid work, while the other performs housework. Yet if one person cleans and the other continuously engages in his/her own interests, the principle of the jointly shared responsibility is challenged. Simultaneously, the experience of being together and having an equal relationship is also threatened. All couple types, even the ones who accept the notion of sameness, emphasise the importance of displaying a jointly shared responsibility. As long as each person's efforts are believed to serve the common good, large discrepancies in work efforts can be accepted, and the parties can uphold their perception of being equal (see also Júlíusdóttir 1993: 168). This is radically different from the sameness principle, which is a method of offsetting individual efforts, needs and interests against each other in the striving for a balance.

The norm of a jointly shared responsibility thus emphasises how important it is that both parties display a priority for the common good. Both parties are meant to take mutual needs into account, that of the self and the other. When the division of labour is suffused with this principle, it is experienced as fair and equal, regardless of whether the parties perform similar amounts of housework or not. The justice principle applied here is not based on sameness, but on needs. Group cohesion is the central issue. In terms of the discussion of Chapter 3, focus here is on the 'communal sharing' relationship.

If this relationship type and its justice principles are challenged openly by one party, the other party will question the division of labour applied and begin to measure the efforts made by the individuals.

Dividing up labour according to the pleasure principle

Experiences of pleasure and displeasure are recurring themes in the rationales that are provided for each type of labour division. The pleasure principle plays a significant role in the division of the labour between the spouses. It also seems to be important in terms of perceptions of justice and injustice, as well as in judgements regarding the equality of the division.

Household labour is to a certain extent described in terms of duties, chores which have to be done, and therefore is easily associated with displeasure. Both women and men regard large parts of household labour as boring, unpleasant and hard work. This could be a reason why divisions made according to the pleasure principle are so significant. Another reason of similar importance is surely that people strive for pleasure, performing acts of satisfaction – also in the household. One woman declares that justice in her view is 'doing what you like'. One husband claims that his and his wife's division of labour is fair because they split the boring work and perform the fun work together. Other interviewees express similar trains of thought:

> We should share certain boring tasks more often.

> You should share the work so that each person has different tasks, split the heavy and the easy, the boring and the nice.

Certain tasks are regarded as more fun compared to others. In the couples of our study, we have not been able to discern any characteristically gender-based preferences. In one of the families, the husband and the wife cook food approximately as many times a week as each other, and the occasion is largely determined by their varying work hours. The husband often cooks at the weekend, because he enjoys it. It is not unusual for men to cook, if they think it is fun. In another family, the husband prepares the weekend meals, and the wife does the cooking for the rest of the week. They always prepare the Friday festive meals together. The husband says: 'I like preparing food, and I will do it when I get a chance.' In some families, the women do all of the shopping, because they think it is 'great fun'. One of them describes it as 'somewhat of a hobby to keep track of prices . . . so I have taken it upon myself to do it.'

Displeasure associated with certain tasks can lead to attempts to transfer them to the partner. The husband who finds it awkward to speak on the phone leaves it to the wife. The wife who hates cleaning lets her husband do it. One strategy of handling disagreeable activities is to split them down the middle. In one family where doing the dishes is regarded as an unpleasant task, a strict calendar rota has been applied to divide up the chores. Every family member is expected to do the dishes as many times a week. Another strategy is to carry out unpleasant work together, which could lead to the inclusion of an element of pleasure to the activities – through the togetherness. Yet another way of handling boring tasks is to carry them out so badly that the other party takes over. This strategy, however, is associated with conflicts and quarrels, thus adding another element of displeasure.

Feelings of pleasure and displeasure in regards to certain tasks are relevant when judging equality and justice. In one couple, both parties maintain that the husband performs most chores. However, the husband does not experience this as unjust, because he is not performing any disagreeable work, 'since I don't think that anything I need to do is boring.' As long as he likes performing the work, he can have a heavier workload without experiencing it as unfair. A similar argument about the relationship between work, pleasure and justice is brought up by a woman who experiences the household work as heavy:

> I think it's mostly the home that is the heavy load, the practical housework. The children stuff is not heavy, that's just fun. It is the home that's boring . . . That's the part that I find most cumbersome. It would have made a difference if I thought it was fun, and then I would surely have done it without saying anything. But since I don't like it, it means that the sacrifice is greater. Kind of like a martyr, sacrificing, I do it although I don't like it.

In the first example, the man lets the pleasure principle compensate for the extra work he does. In the second example, feelings of pleasure could have compensated for the skewed division of labour. Instead, the injustice is worsened by the fact that the tasks are experienced as very dull. The injustice is traced back to the fact that an uneven workload is combined with unpleasant tasks.

In another couple, the husband claims that the division of labour between him and the wife is unjust because he does only the things he likes, while the wife does things that he regards as dull and boring, mainly cleaning and tidying. The wife also argues in terms of pleasure and displeasure when she judges their division of labour. She claims to dislike some of the tasks that the husband performs, such as driving the children to hockey and football tournaments.

> In reality, he takes on a great responsibility. Like the children. He takes them to football and handball, and sometimes it's football and handball all weekend. It takes all day. And then I can't claim to carry a heavy load when I'm at home cleaning for a few hours, while he is at the football field all day in the pouring rain from seven to three with the children.

Instead of standing outside all day, getting wet and cold, she prefers to take care of the cleaning. In her description, an image of rain, nasty weather and discomfort is contrasted to the quiet and calm of the house, where she can clean according to her own discretion. Possibly, she utilises the pleasure principle in order to justify and regulate a feeling of imbalance in their way of dividing the household work.

These examples tell us that feelings of pleasure or displeasure elicited by various household duties are utilised when judging whether the division of labour is balanced, fair or unfair. The pleasure principle is combined with other principles. Time spent on pleasant tasks is not regarded as equal to time spent on disagreeable tasks. Feelings of pleasure compensate for imbalances in terms of time. Displeasure heightens perceptions of imbalance in amount of work carried out, and strengthens the sense of injustice. The different components of time, task, pleasure and displeasure are thus related to one another in an equation of sorts. Arguments led in terms of pleasure and displeasure are led by men as well as women. In this respect, there is no difference between couples who apply different models of labour division.

The significance of preferences and feelings of pleasure and displeasure for the shaping of the division of labour has been given attention by other researchers, such as Ahrne and Roman (1997), but the principle as such has not been subject to deeper discussion. One exception is an Australian study about the organisation of housework among couples with unconventional divisions of labour. The researchers describe their surprise over how openly and frequently the participants spoke about what chores they liked and loathed, and that this affected the division of labour (Goodnow and Bowes 1994). We were also mildly astonished over how common the mentioning of pleasure and displeasure was. This surprise can possibly be explained by the scant space provided by previous research on divisions of household labour to issues of desire.

Being competent

One common reason why a certain division of labour is applied is often that one partner has a greater competence in specific tasks. One of them is simply better at certain things, such as repairs, cooking, planning, effective purchases or administration of the family budget. Issues of competence are sometimes associated with gender; we will return to this issue in the next section.

The competence-based labour divisions are sometimes related to professions, perhaps most clearly when it comes to issues of finance. Men's responsibility for the budget is sometimes motivated by their education in economics. In one case, it was natural that the woman should handle the family finances, since she worked as a cashier at a post office. On the other hand, in another family where the wife also was a cashier, the husband took the responsibility for the finances. Competence gained in the work sphere can sometimes be presented as the reason for a certain division of labour, whereas similar competence in other cases does not have the same effect.

The most common strategy is to let personal qualifications decide. There are examples of men who almost always cook, and the reason given is that they are the better at it. They cook the tastiest food. Women often give that reason, whereas the men themselves motivate it in accordance with the pleasure principle – that they enjoy doing it. We have previously mentioned several examples of women who do all the shopping, including the men's clothes. They justify it by saying that they enjoy it, but they also think that they are better at the task. Their husbands agree and describe them as being extremely good at finding the cheapest and the best, a competence that contributes to some extent of family luxury, despite a limited budget.

When discussing competence, there are two more general lines of argument. One focuses on the advantages in having a specialised division of labour. Just like in professional life, each person does what he or she is best at. Often this is the case of utilising a competence that one already possesses. 'Splitting the work according to each person's competence' is regarded by one woman as an important main principle in the division of labour that they have given shape to. 'Each one takes care of their special area, i.e. what they are best at,' one man states about their established division of labour. This principle may of course have awkward consequences for the woman if the man is not accomplished in *any* household work. In divisions of labour based on competence, people specialise in performing different tasks. According to a classic, sociological line of argument, this would lead to enhancing the parties' mutual dependence. The family cohesion would be strengthened through specialisation of labour. Another perspective in social science emphasises that specialisation brings effectiveness, and in every social organisation including the household group, a specialisation that follows competence is thus created (Becker 1993).

An alternative line of argument adopted by the couples is the will to counteract specialisation. The aim is for both to develop an 'all-round' ability that each person should be able to carry out all tasks in the home. Some men in particular emphasise the importance of this. 'There is no area I can't manage or that she can't manage.' 'You should be able to manage most things, and not refrain from doing housework because you are unable,' another man points out.

It is said to be good for the relationship to be able to do things together. Performing tasks together, such as cooking, cleaning and car or boat maintenance, creates good collaboration and a special kind of joy. In this line of argument, the emphasis is not on established competencies, but rather on the ability to acquire new skills. Based on this line of thought, this would imply that the spouses are not co-dependent, since each person could manage on his/her own. However, the advocates for the all-round competence instead emphasise the strengthening of the feelings of togetherness and solidarity.

Competence, as in one party being better at performing a task than the other, is a way of motivating a certain division of labour. This motivation is rarely used when the parties are judging whether the division of labour is fair or equal. Preferences, i.e. pleasure and displeasure, seem to be significantly more determining in such judgements.

Acknowledging a traditional gender division of labour

The significance of gender for division of labour in the home has been demonstrated in countless studies, and appears also in this investigation. In couples where the woman performs typical 'female' chores and the male performs 'male' tasks, gender is of course relevant. But what significance is attributed to gender in families where at least one partner wishes for a gender non-specific organisation? How do women and men talk about gender in these circumstances?

It is rare that a certain division of labour is directly motivated in terms of gender. Personal qualifications or preferences are instead mentioned. Yet, it is still apparent that gender gives structure to the division of labour, although it is not referred to explicitly. This becomes particularly clear in two types of activities. One concerns repairs in the home, which is regarded as a typical male duty. The other is the ability to predict and plan, which is described as a female thing throughout. Decoration, 'adornment' and renewing the home are also part of the female sphere. These patterns are obvious among those who have a gender-traditional division of labour, but are also applicable to the remaining couples. How are these gender-based types of labour division motivated?

Here we shall report only on what the men are expected to do, namely repairs, carpentry and car maintenance. These activities are presented as strongly gender assigned, i.e. they belong to the men's sphere of activities whether they like it or not.

In an attempt to clarify who does what tasks best, one woman concludes that she is best at planning, and her husband is best at all things technical. He repairs things, refurbishes, and fixes the car. She maintains that his handiness fulfils a practical function in her life, but she also maintains that his skill represents something attractive in her view. This competence carries erotic overtones, and thus transcends the purely practical view. She says that her husband takes care of everything to do with the car:

I think that's important, because I would not like to get stuck in and learn it. Because my husband does it. He's good with those things, and he is my man. So in a strange way, he can. And I think it's very good, I couldn't . . . I would not have chosen a man with two left hands . . . The worst thing I know is guys who have to try everything and never succeed. I think those guys are unattractive. I'd rather they'd say: 'I'm an intellectual, I don't lift a finger'. Those who think that they can and try, and no good comes out of it. It is really unattractive. I think he is very attractive as a man, because he is good at the things he does.

Even if this woman expresses the connection between technical ability, masculinity and attraction with unique clarity, other women also express similar trains of thought, albeit in vaguer terms. One woman maintains that her husband is important to her. He is the one who takes care of reparations, simply because he is a man. This type of handiness seems to represent a vital part of masculinity to her:

My husband has never demanded that I do anything special because I am a woman. On the other hand, I might have, because he is a man in a different way, and he should be handy. Luckily he is, like with repairs.

Masculinity–handiness (carpentry and refurbishment) seems to configure a cohesive thought Gestalt. There are clear demands on the man, tasks that he must perform in order to be a man. In some cases, aspects of attraction are not dominant in the women's statements, but rather the demands on male handiness. For instance, one of the women expresses mainly irritation at her husband's dislike of fixing broken objects:

He knows so much. He is incredibly practical, but I think it is horribly dull, so those are things I can become very irritated with – things not being fixed. I am no good at all fixing things. And it's the same with the car, too. I think you can do that, can't you, you know the car. He can take it apart completely, that he can do, but he doesn't do it unless there is an absolute emergency. Only when it is dead and doesn't run. Then there are little things that are not right in it for a long time, and that I become ticked off over.

The husband describes an almost insurmountable resistance towards fixing things that are broken. 'I become almost paralysed, actually, when there is something I must do.' Possibly, this feeling of paralysis could be related to the demands the wife makes, making him feel coerced to display masculinity.

Sometimes, the outliers or 'deviants' can make patterns appear clearer. In one family, the man differs from most men by almost never fixing things that are broken. He also believes that 'changing light bulbs and put up curtain rails', what the wife does in their home, is 'more of a male thing'. The wife does not comment on the light bulbs or the curtain rails, but is very clear about her irritation over the fact that she is always the one who has to remove the bathtub front when the bathroom is being cleaned. One could speculate if her anger is related to a feeling of injustice in the allocation of boring tasks, or if it is related to her always having to perform typically male tasks. In another couple, the woman refers to herself as 'deviant', because she is the one who cleans the sewer pipes and deals with technical things.

Men's dominance in the technical field is of course an effect of gender socialisation. A complementary explanation is related to the desire to distinguish between the genders. Femininity as an identity requires an opposite in masculinity, and vice versa. This means that the creation of gender identity requires the difference. However, the project of equality requires sameness. There is a clear tension between these strivings (see Bjerrum Nielsen and Rudberg 1994; Thagaard 1996). 'Making gender' requires the upholding of masculinity and femininity. The tendency to adhere to specific male and female zones can thus be interpreted as a way of maintaining these distinctions. Male dominance in terms of technology, refurbishment and repairs is hence not only a practical solution to a practical problem, and not only a consequence of gender socialisation. It is equally important to uphold gender differences. Male handiness is given an erotic attribution that can be viewed from this angle of interpretation.

Gender is rarely used to motivate a certain division of labour. One reason could be that our interview did not ask the question from that viewpoint. Another reason could be that these arguments are not regarded as legitimate when talking about fairness and equality.

Three approaches to the division of labour and gender equality

Following our presentation of different principles utilised to motivate the division of labour and judging its justice, we will return to the approaches that were presented in the introduction of the chapter. We differentiated between three ways of speaking about the division of labour. One way was to create agreements, a kind of contract; another circulated around a spontaneously emerged division of labour based on the needs of both parties; and in the third way, division of labour was regarded as self-emergent, as something that just appeared. Below, we will provide a more detailed description of their implications.

Contract-oriented division of labour and equality

Contract-oriented couples create explicit agreements about who is responsible for different chores in the home. Some chores are scheduled, and each person knows his or her responsibility. Also the children can have explicit rules for what they should do.

In one of the couples, both the woman and the man emphasise the importance of having a clear and specific division of labour. In his view, conflicts regarding division of labour are practical – you have to look at it from a practical viewpoint and find a solution. The solution for this couple has implied compromise and reaching agreements about how things are to be done. Each person knows exactly what chores he or she (and the children) are meant to carry out. It happens that the rules are bent, but clear rules should always be in place in terms of the labour division.

The notion of equality in this family is primarily associated with sameness. Fairness results when all parties do as much. This value can be combined with e.g. pleasure and displeasure in more complex calculations. An example of this type of calculation mentioned previously was the agreement on the cleaning. Both parties dislike cleaning, but the husband carries out the larger share of this work. In this sense, there is an element of sacrifice on his behalf. However, he cleans less frequently and less meticulously than his wife wishes for, which she must accept in exchange for not having to do as much cleaning.

In the contract-oriented way of reasoning about division of labour, the couples have an outspoken feeling for contractual thinking and for agreements based on the relative advantages of each party. The relationship between giving and taking is important, and factors of not only time but also pleasure and displeasure are weighed into the calculation. Justice is about beneficial settlements for both, and if they are reached, whatever you put in you get out. Contract allocations regarding the household work are clear, and have a specialisation based on a combination of competence and preference. Each person develops a competence in a different area, the degree of specialisation is high and, to a certain extent, the division of labour transcends gender order.

According to the contract-oriented view of division of labour in the home, agreements and allocations between the parties is something positive. Clear expressions of 'You do that' and 'I do this' create orderly structures and the number of conflicts is fewer. Allocations can vary over time and be renegotiated. The notion of justice orbits around sameness or proportionality, with two relatively autonomous 'egos' striving for sameness in order to reach balance, weighing each effort against the other. In relation to Fiske's (1991, 1992) reasoning (see Chapter 3) it can be seen as a social relation characterised by an equal balance or calculation.

Needs-oriented division of labour and equality

Both spouses in needs-oriented couples claim that the household work is not formally divided, but runs 'naturally'. There is never a need to agree on who does what, since both do what needs to be done in the home. The person who gets home first does the shopping, cooking, laundry, and cares for the children etc. Chores are often carried out together. Recurring phrases are 'What needs to be done is done' or 'We do many things together.' Furthermore, 'We don't have yours and mine, but we do what is needed. And often we do things together.'

The central principle for couples with this orientation is that of shared responsibility, not sameness in time or effort. Pleasure and displeasure rule the development of specialisation to a limited extent. Primarily, the present needs direct both parties' efforts. Doing things together, not in the least the dull tasks, has a value in itself. There are no schedules, no clear and distinctive allocations of work, no chores that belong to either party, but demands on both partners to make sure that common needs are seen to. The main criterion is that both have the competence to tend to all tasks in a home. Circumstance, place and time determine who does what. The aim is that both develop a competence for all household work. Thus, there are no gender-specific tasks, and the level of specialisation is low.

In descriptions of the division of labour, attention is brought to its 'spontaneous' emergence. This is also the case with equality. The implicit message is that it should be that way. You do not bargain or negotiate a division of labour; it should emerge spontaneously in that both address common needs.

The needs-oriented approach does not accept divisions of mine and yours. Instead, the parties' mutual dependence is emphasised, and that 'we are the ones who do' something, together or separately. If present needs and circumstances determine, both parties must be observant and flexible to adapt to them. The needs-oriented approach thus places great demands on the parties in a relationship. The thought of weighing efforts against each other is unacceptable, as is the conscious striving towards reaching balance. Gender is not attributed with a decisive influence in the repertoire of activities. The model of social relationships that is advocated is very much associated with 'communal sharing' in Fiske's typology, with a concept of justice that is expressly needs based.

Gender-based division of labour and equality

The third variation presented here involves a division of labour regulated according to women's and men's different qualities and obligations. Women in couples who have a characteristically gender-based division of labour can say, 'We are quite divided into the feminine and masculine'. They refer to equality 'the old-fashioned way'. The division of labour is claimed to have emerged and ended up a certain way. Different chores in the household 'just carry on'. No agreements have ever been made regarding allocations and turn-taking such as 'This week you clean because you did it last week.'

In these couples, there are clear allocations of what each person should do in everyday life. The specialisation stretches quite far, and is gender based. Gender boundaries may, however, be transcended, when the woman does 'male things' such as changing light bulbs and putting up a shelf on the wall. It happens that the husband cooks dinners on special occasions, 'treating' the wife and children to something festive. She then feels courted and he feels as if he is courting her, simply because the fixed, established gender roles are transcended. Performing the same is not a high priority, and the competence is associated with gender without reflection. It is important to both partners that the responsibility for the family and the common good is shared.

Couples with this division of labour can see themselves as equal, even if the argument in favour of this has a defensive character. It takes the shape of a defence for the notion that also this kind of division of labour can be 'equal'.

The foundation for this type of gender-differentiated labour division is that men and women act within their respective 'spheres'. Labour specialisation is clear, and determined by the supposition that the genders have particular knowledge. Each sphere is necessary for the jointly shared, but the specific tasks in the respective spheres are gender determined. Since gender determines the task, they are negotiable to a small extent. 'It just ended up that way', as many of the involved express it. The sameness notion is not adequate in these circumstances, nor is the notion that each person could be responsible for all the needs of the family. Justice is connected to each person performing his or her acts within the gender-defined sphere. It is a relationship that is strictly gender structured, and that rests on an inbuilt authority order.

Ideals and practice

We would like to point out that it is our intention to present the three models of division of labour as ideal types. We disregard the fact that contract-oriented couples can also have significant elements of needs-orientation, and that needs-oriented couples also have contract-oriented elements. In other words, we describe tendencies that could be more or less dominating in different couples. Occasionally, individuals in the same couple also differ. One may want to have clear divisions and agreements, whereas the other resists dissecting everyday life in that way.

With reference to Kellerhal and colleagues' (1988, 1997) research results (see Chapter 4), we can expect that the respective priorities for 'agreements' and 'needs' occur in accordance with social class or education, status and occupational field. Is this visible in our material? We can confirm that for all couples with a contract-oriented view of division of labour, the spouses are very similar in terms of education, income and occupation. The women whose salaries are slightly higher than the men's also belong to this category. In couples with a needs-oriented division of labour, we find couples with similar occupation and incomes, but there are also examples of large income differences in this group. Overall, this material is not suitable to draw such conclusions.

However, there is another, more distinctive aspect to consider – the relationship between ideals and practice. Clearly, a contract-oriented division of labour is dominant among women who have fought to achieve a more equal division of labour. In the agreements, they see a guarantee for a fairer division of labour, as could their husbands. Men as well as women in couples with a traditional division of labour perceive it as having emerged by itself. Couples who employ a mutual collaboration predominantly have what we refer to as a needs-based orientation.

The question is then – what role do the ideals play for the practice that is developed? There is not a great difference between ideals and practice among the women who have fought for an equal division of labour. They have attained a model consisting of agreements that are adhered to, and view this as the ideal division of labour. A needs-based view dominates among couples who cooperate in the household labour and have no conflicts on the issue. We can draw the significant, yet not so sensational conclusion that the practice is probably relevant to how the ideals are shaped. Women, who have had to fight for an equal division of labour to reach the ideal through agreements, view it as the ideal form. Without the necessity to overcome resistance, the needs-based orientation would have been the given ideal. In other words: ideals are neither stabile nor independent of circumstances. They are changeable and influenced by individual and jointly shared experiences.

However, there are also examples of clear opposition between expressed ideals and the existing practice of labour division. In these cases, the ideals have not been adapted to the practice. This is the case with women who are not very successful in their fight for an equal division of labour. These women want agreements and allocations, but this is not realised in the practical everyday life. Their ideals act as a driving force in the attempts at mobilising a practical change. There are also other examples of opposing ideals and practices. For instance, women who have become discontented with the established traditional division of labour pose a needs-oriented ideal against a practice that is lacking in that respect. The longing for a needs-oriented practice is striking. Yet, the expectation that it should arise spontaneously, by itself, simultaneously seems to create obstacles for change. One of these women says that equality is important, but not if it is reached through directing and coercion:

> It shouldn't be forced, but happen naturally. But I don't know if there are such relationships, where it happens naturally. I don't know. I count on the fact that – equality for me is that you should not force things. You shouldn't shape it should just be, you shouldn't have to work on it because then it turns out wrong. Fighting for it makes it wrong. Women's groups and suchlike . . . no, no. That makes it wrong; you direct too much, I can't handle that. Then the whole purpose is kind of wrong.

Equality is almost described as utopia in this case. It is a desired object, but presented as something that must arise by itself, and not be forced. Other women also have a similar view. Help, when given by the other, must be self-started, otherwise forget about it. One woman says that her husband is driving her crazy because he rarely helps out in the home, but she still does not want to ask for help:

I guess it's that I don't think you should ask for things. I'm afraid to nag if I keep on asking. I think it should be a given that you do certain things. But it isn't, and then I'd rather let it go and do it myself.

These women are not satisfied with their situation, but see no solution. Their approach to negotiations and agreements is insecure and trembling, perhaps due to prior failure. Their ambivalence can also be seen as reflecting a betrayal towards the notion of mutuality. Having to ask for something that is perceived as given, can also lead to subordination. Having to approach the other with dependence, and wondering whether the other could please help, is subordinating. Refusing to ask for help can become a way of avoiding subordination. It is also a way of solving the problem of the absent signs of love stemming from the lack of an expressed will to cooperate. If you do not nag, the absence becomes less clearly demonstrated. As long as perceptions of mutuality are important in the economy of love, it may be better not to make demands. 'If it isn't a given to the other person, then let it be, you don't want it.'

Some reflections

Theories of social psychology state that human beings in social situations that do not have objective criteria for comparison tend to only compare themselves with their peers. As pointed out by Van Yperen and Buunk (1994), comparisons between men's and women's work efforts thus become pointless in societies or social groups with a strict gender-based division of labour. Women in this case tend to compare themselves to other women in the group rather than with the men, who represent a completely different category. Comparisons between the genders become relevant when men and women are active on the same arena. Questions regarding what they get out of the interaction with each other will then become meaningful. In modern marriages, social comparisons between the parties become important issues. Consequently, the type of justice that compares input with output becomes relevant (Van Yperen and Buunk 1994).

In this chapter, we have seen examples of some of the implications that the concept of equality can have for people – and thus far, only in the issues of labour division. We have witnessed that people in their perceptions of justice apply several different principles that sometimes weave together in an intricate pattern. We have described three equality ideals and patterns of labour division that seem to be connected with various constellations of these principles. The contract-oriented ideal is open to comparisons of input and output, in line with Van Yperen and Buunk's (1994) argument. Comparing the size and volume of the other person's efforts appears to be reasonable in this ideal. The concept of a fair order that rests on sameness in effort is as reasonable. Such comparisons are irrelevant in the needs-oriented ideal. It applies a different equality concept, another view of what constitutes a fair and just order, with emphasis on a needs-based justice and jointly shared responsibilities. The gender-based ideal applies a relatively fixed and categorical justice concept, where each person fulfils his or her duties according to status.

The concept of equality, as applied to division of labouring family life, hosts a great deal of complexity. In Chapter 7, we will look at other aspects of everyday life, and will thus come across other implications of this concept.

Chapter 7

Sharing and allocating money

How are incomes and expenses allocated in contemporary families where both parties are in waged labour? Are negotiations about finances carried out in the open, free of conflict, or are they associated with substantial clashes? Themes of money allocation to the common good and the individual give a concrete expression of the internal relationships between the spouses from the reciprocity and justice perspectives. In cases where both spouses have paid work, each of them contributes to the common household and the children. Most probably, each of the spouses has an opinion of how much money should be set aside for the common good, what the children's costs should be, and what is fair in different types of allocations to the children and between the partners in the relationship. Money carries a symbolic value not only for mutuality and togetherness in the family, but also for the independence of each person in the couple relationship. The relationship between the common budget and the space for personal consumption is about power and dependence. Financial dependence is viewed as an important cause of women's subordination in families, although it is not the only cause (Roman 1999). It is therefore interesting to study how women's own incomes influence the division of power between the genders in couple relationships.

What does the law say about shared and separate finances in couple relationships? In a Swedish marriage, according to marital law, both parties are obliged to support each other according to ability. This obligation does not include cohabiting partners who are not married. Furthermore, husbands and wives have a right to know about each other's incomes. This is not the case for cohabiting partners. In cohabiting families, the main principle is the financial independence of each party. In marriages, the main principle is joint finances. By signing a prenuptial agreement, the spouses can secure their rights to property and valuables in the home, and thereby differentiate the individual economy from the joint finances. The legislation thus carries the message of a normative ideal of a jointly shared economy. In cohabiting couples (married and unmarried), the common practice is to consider the finances as joint, and that they should be divided equally if the parties divorce (Agell 1998).

In a study on how couples divided their finances, it was found that all parties advocated for having equal standards (Nyman 2002). This result appeared to be valid in our study, too. But, similarly to Nyman's study, the practice did not coincide fully with the ideals. Certainly, the kind of economy relevant to traditional nuclear families, where the husband earns money and the wife takes care of the children and family, is not very common in Sweden any more. However, more married and cohabiting women (40 per cent) compared to men (25 per cent) felt that they could not afford things that they deemed vital.[1] In the same study, it was revealed that more women (49 per cent) than men (37 per cent) perceived themselves as *not* having money to spend on themselves.

Money: control and management

One aspect of the allocation of power over money is the organisation of how resources and assets are administered and controlled in families. A major study on this topic was made in Great Britain in the early 1980s. Four different styles were discerned: a so-called housewife management style, where the husband hands all his income to the wife, who in turn takes care of the household budget and consumption. This style was primarily applied in households with small incomes, and where virtually all the money that came in was spent. The second style consisted of the husband giving pocket money to the wife, but retaining control, and his spouse had to ask for money for her own and the family's consumption. In the third housekeeping style, the husband gave a fixed sum to the wife for the household consumption, but took care of the remaining amount. The fourth style implied joint management, where both partners were responsible for the majority of the finances in the household (Pahl 1989).

In a comparative study of Swedish and British families from the 1990s, it was found that the first three styles hardly exist in Sweden, which is mainly due to the fact that both parties undertake paid work. According to the study, joint management was by far the most common type of administration – 82 per cent of the Swedish families in the study had some form of joint pooling. In Great Britain, joint pooling was applied by approximately half of the studied families (Roman and Vogler 1999). Another Swedish study shows that 90 per cent of the households applied some form of joint pooling (Nyman 2002).

What is meant by joint management of the household economy? Shared administration can be practised in many ways. In Nyman's study, the participants displayed numerous variations and combinations of separate and shared finances. In the study, measurements were made of each party in a couple as to perceptions of the allocation of money, decision-making on the use of money and satisfaction of the applied order, as well as what was known about the other person's consumption (Nyman 2002). In the comparative study of British and Swedish families, three variations of the joint pooling were discerned. The main criteria used by the researchers in order to establish patterns consisted of a question on who had the last word in terms of the economy in the household.[2]

The first model was based on the woman having the main responsibility (27 per cent in Sweden), the second model was based on the man having the main responsibility (35 per cent in Sweden), and the third model was based on joint management. Joint management was applied by approximately 20 per cent (n = 1162) in both countries. The model of male main responsibility for the economy was the predominant model in both Sweden and Great Britain in households where the husband earned more money than the wife (Nyman 2002).

One way of organising the economy is to split expenses. In the study from 1992 that formed the basis for the study presented in this book,[3] questions were asked on this theme: 25 per cent of the women and 19 per cent of the men replied that they had split expenses. The expenses managed by the women were food (70 per cent), childcare (42 per cent), children's clothing and other daily expenses (82 per cent) and own clothes (77 per cent). Men's expenses were predominantly concerned with own clothes (73 per cent), the car (83 per cent) and residential (85 per cent). These figures show that different expenses in the household are gender assigned, the women managing the expenses of the children, food and clothing – which they are responsible for from day to day – whereas the men's expenses are mainly concerned with capital goods.

Ways of measuring joint management can vary, and thus provide different answers. This is associated with the organisation of the economy in the household being a very complex issue, which in turn implies that perceptions of money as shared or separate can be very subtle. Both Nyman (2002) and our own study exemplify this, and the results of the latter will be demonstrated below.

Joint, split and separated – a few concepts

This study includes detailed scrutiny of the internal economic allocation of spouses by way of several types of questions regarding the organisation of household and individual finances. The guiding theme in the questions regarded the differentiation between individual economic freedom and control over consumption and savings for joint and personal needs. The spouses' incomes, property, accounts and debts have been taken into account. We have differentiated between what is individual and what is jointly shared. In terms of consumption, questions were asked about how the division between the spouses was made in the household and in personal consumption. Furthermore, questions were asked regarding the management of bills, in other words, who makes the payment and makes sure it is on time.

For each couple, a schematic overview over their economic allocation was made (see example in Table 1).

We also utilised *statements* (vignettes) to introduce a conversation with the interviewees regarding their perceptions of different principles for separate and joint issues in terms of the household budget. The purpose of these questions

Table 1 Example of economic splitting within couples

	Property	Household consumption	Personal consumption	Household savings	Personal savings	Income relation between spouses	Management
Woman	Summer house, co-owned with brother	Fixed bills	Own cash	Her income for the children, savings account	Separate savings account	She earns more	She manages the bills
Man	Boat	Ongoing expenses	Own cash	His incomes, savings account	Separate savings account	He earns marginally less	
Both	House, caravan				Un-expected expenses		

was to find out what is regarded as *ideal and morally correct* when it comes to economic division into joint and separate. One of the vignettes tells of a couple with a partially shared economy. The woman earns more than the man, and they share expenses equally, which means that she has more left over for personal consumption compared to him. The interviewed couples are asked to judge whether they think this is an acceptable principle of division. Another vignette tells of a woman in a couple who is given cash as a gift from a relative. She wants to use the money to travel by herself. The question is whether she has a moral right to use the money for her personal purposes and make that decision on her own.

Furthermore, we asked the respondents to think about their own attitudes concerning saving and consumption, and to compare these perceptions with that of their partner. Questions were also asked regarding decisions and conflicts regarding economic issues and *how they perceive economic equality*. The vantage points for economic negotiation can also be dependent on relatives, economic transfers between them and adult children as well as children in the family. We asked if such situations apply or have applied in the past, and how this support has been perceived by the partner.

In the analysis of the replies, three analytical dimensions were discerned. The first dimension is the relationship between *ideals and practice*. This refers to outspoken ideals, what is thought to be morally right in allocation of money into separate and joint spheres, and whether it is congruous with the practice adopted by the couple.[4]

Joint–separate is the second dimension. What does a joint or separate economy on a practical level imply? 'Separate economy' is in opposition to joint economy and implies 'yours and mine'. This could mean that each person handles his or her own accounts, and the other person has no access or insight into how these monies are kept and consumed.

'Allocation' in this context refers to the money being divided into different accounts, how the accounts are topped up and what purpose they fill. *Practically*, the division means that the couple has some kind of agreement regarding how expenses, costs and savings are to be managed. This concerns how different accounts have been opened for joint and separate consumption, the division ownership of properties such as the house, car, summer house and savings in personal accounts. *Morally*, it concerns what the division means to the couple relationship, the *symbolic significance in the togetherness of the couple and the division of power in the couple.*

Control–administration constitutes the third dimension. In this context, control refers to decision-making regarding how money is distributed and spent. This is about how money is managed in the family, and the influence over joint and separate consumption. Furthermore, it concerns decisions on purchases, expenses as well as setting an upper limit of expenditure, and how any surpluses should be used. Control is not the same as administration of money. Administration here refers to making sure that all expenses and bills are met. This implies saving and making sure that cash is available for purchases. This is work, a responsibility that holds one accountable, but does not necessarily provide control or power.

Allocation and distribution of money: empirical examples

Different models emerge in the analysis of couples' organisation of their finances. As mentioned above, joint pooling has several implications. The couples frequently advocated the principle of having joint finances, but in practice it was revealed that divisions of various kinds were often made within the framework of what was considered to be the joint economy. Behind this dissonance were different principles of justice and togetherness. In our material, there are also examples of couples where perceptions of ideals were dissimilar, and the practice ended up in a kind of combination of joint and separate. Below, we will present a few examples to illustrate how different couples argued what was ideal and suitable in practice in their relationship. The examples are chosen because they represent the patterns we discerned, and because they display the further reaches in the organisation of the relationship between the joint and the separate according to the dimensions described above.

Separate economy as ideal and practice

Both partners in the couples who represent the management style described here had a similar professional education and both were full-time workers. He earned more than she did.

Allocations

This example is a couple who, like most couples, have a joint account for fixed joint expenses, and separate accounts for personal consumption. Both saved approximately equal amounts in separate pension funds. Furthermore, they saved equal amounts in an account that existed for unforeseen expenses or larger purchases. The child allowance was put into a separate account, from which expenses for the child were withdrawn. They have joint ownership of their property. The man had separate savings capital, the woman did not.

Deposits into the joint accounts were made according to the principle of equal payments. Since the woman had a lower income than the man, she had fewer surpluses for her own consumption. The man sometimes covered the day-to-day expenses, since his earnings were greater.

Control

In this couple, the husband administered the budget. The wife participated in paying the bills, since she also wanted to be involved in the joint economy. They had agreed on the financial allocation that was in place, both saying that they wished to retain control over what was in their separate accounts. Her opinion was that if they had a joint account that included personal expenses, it would be necessary to check each other's outgoings on a continuous basis. This would bring insecurity in relation to what existed in the account. The absence of control would create this insecurity. It was the man who took the initiative to open separate accounts:

> He wants to know how much he has left so that I don't come along and say that I've made withdrawals from your account, now you don't have as much left as you think you did. I went along with that and thought it was good.

Right to personal money

The partners had different standards, since the wife's income was lower, and she also had debts that she was repaying on her own. Despite their differences in personal standards, they both approved of their model. The woman thought that it provided her with her own economic space. For example, if she wished to make a purchase for herself, she withdrew the money from her own account, if it contained any money, otherwise she would borrow from the joint account and repay when her next salary cheque arrived. Or she would postpone the purchase until her salary was paid.

The husband claimed that he did not think that any other model would be possible for him:

> Well, I have to have it like this. I don't want to share money with anyone. We share that which must be joint, and then we have our own money. She doesn't ask me if she wants to buy something and I don't ask her. Then you have to be responsible and feel that you can't buy a new aerobics outfit if the money is gone and you need to buy food and only half the month has gone by.

He was aware that they had different limitations for personal consumption, but claimed that it wasn't his fault, that the problem was her low salary. She had shared her husband's viewpoint regarding her low salary. With a higher salary, she would have higher limits for her personal consumption.

Ideal and practice

The ideal model was not applied to its full extent, since the husband at times covered day-to-day joint expenses. She did not adhere to the model strictly either, since she sometimes used her separate account to cover joint expenses. This was particularly the case with the food. Not drawing a strict line between her own assets and the joint consumption implied a certain amount of pressure in terms of her own consumption. She felt that she must hold back, being afraid that the joint assets would suffer. She could feel guilty if she went shopping for herself. In such situations, she would ask the husband for advice, and if he approved, she would make the purchase. In practice, this meant that the husband was given control over her personal consumption. She told the interviewer:

> Sometimes I can feel guilty if I have bought something for myself, despite the fact that I have my own account. I feel as though I cannot spend my whole salary privately. What should we live off then? It should be spent on food and the likes, too. You know approximately how much you have left to spend. If there is something that I need, he actually says, 'Of course you should buy it.' If he says that, it is not hard, otherwise I can get a guilty conscience. If he supports me, then I'd gladly do it.

Her governance over her personal consumption, coupled with her husband's relative economic freedom, in practice resulted in him having the economic power in the family. Both were of the opinion that they viewed money differently. He wanted to spend and she wanted to hold back. They had discussions about how expenses should be prioritised, in which she tried to express an opinion on his personal spending in relation to the jointly shared. In these discussions, she would often have to cede, since he would use his own account for that spending. 'It always ends up all right,' she claims, 'he takes it from his own account and treats himself.' He admitted openly that he had the economic power, but justified it with his higher salary.

Summary

Three couples applied this principle for the separate and jointly shared. The men in this category earned more and spent more on themselves, which meant that the spouses had different standards in their lives. The reasoning behind this was to enable a differentiation between yours and mine and the jointly shared, and that it was important that one party did not consume at the other party's expense.

Male control of all spending

Both partners in this couple were workers and had a similar education. The husband earned more than the wife but the difference was not large. She worked 80 per cent of full time. Both partners asserted that their relationship was equal.

Allocations

In the couple used as an example for this style, there was no joint account, but the divisions consisted of specified costs being withdrawn from the separate personal accounts.

The wife paid for the children's clothing, food and living costs (mortgage payments). Her entire income was spent on joint costs. The husband paid for all recurring bills, certain living costs and insurances. The child allowance was put into a separate account. He had savings in a household account, but he also had personal savings derived from revenues from other activities. They jointly owned a flat and he owned a car.

Control

In this couple, the husband had complete control over the budget, including the wife's expenses. She administered the bills, i.e. prepared them for him to sign – including her personal bills. In other words, she organised everything and made sure the bills were paid for. She argued that they should have a joint economy, but the husband was against it, since he wanted to control the household finances, including her expenses.

Right to personal money

This model yields unequal scope for economic action. The wife had to ask her husband for money for her personal expenditures. She claimed, 'It is not a problem', even though it allowed him to interfere in her judgements about what to buy. Rather, she had the impression that he was generous and always gave her money when she needed it. He was under the same impression: 'I am a very kind person, so generally speaking she gets what she wants.' However, in cases where he did not approve of what she wanted to buy, she had to ask several times. In the end, he usually would cave in. He explained:

> Of course she can have money from me. If she doesn't have money and wants to buy stuff, then I give it to her so that she can buy it. But there must not be any unnecessary impulse purchases. Stuff like that. Then she has to pay for it.

She kept her consumption on a low level:

> 'No, I rarely do that [buy things for herself] . . . often, if I go downtown or so . . . Maybe you have a gift voucher or so when it's your birthday, you have to buy clothes or so, then I come home with something for my daughter or husband, presents, clothes and buy very little for myself – the most necessary.'

She did not mind him saving his own money – she regarded it as reasonable since she claimed that 'he is very economically minded and trades shares and the like . . . But the money that he earns will be spent for joint purposes anyhow'.

Ideal and practice

Both partners claimed that it was important that they had the same living standards, in the sense that one of them should not have more personal money to spend than the other. However, the woman and the man in this couple had different opinions on the ideal. The woman wanted a joint economy: 'I mean if you're married you share everything. Who can spare fifty pounds each month is less important. The one with more money can do that, so to speak.' He claimed: 'I don't want to merge my money with her income and have a joint pool; I want to have control over my money'. But he also said 'My money and my money? It is spent on her any way.' *He expressed an opinion that he had power and wanted to have power but in the end he spent his money on jointly shared items, not for his personal needs.*

This attitude was also present in their reflections on the vignette about the gift. She argued that the right to use the gift was conditional and required the positive consent of the husband. She claimed that she would never have undertaken a journey on her own and argued that the money gift should have been used jointly. He argued that the use of the gift was conditional and had to be 'earned'. It should also be related to other needs of the family: 'It could be the case in a family that there are other needs that are more important than her travelling on her own.'

In terms of economic sharing, this couple represents a classic male-dominated style, an 'authority ranking' model, with the husband claiming the right to have full control over money and exchange. The wife regarded their relationship as equal, since her husband did not dominate her and because they shared domestic work without her needing to nag. Her view was that equality could not be judged in terms of principles of similarity. Women and men are not similar. He expressed a similar view.

Summary

Six of the interviewed couples displayed a similar pattern. The characteristics of this group were that the men had more spending power, often due to their significantly higher salaries and personal savings. The women did not have much left over for their personal consumption – either because their model of allocation did not leave any scope for it, or because they contributed more to the recurring joint costs. The men had more power than the women in this group, but it was often the women who planned purchases and administered the bill payments. All women in this category claimed to get guilty consciences when they bought something for themselves.

Joint pooling as ideal and practice

In this couple both partners had a similar education. He earned a little more than she did. Both worked full time.

Allocations

The couple representing this model had a joint account which paid for all current expenses. Money was transferred monthly from their salary account into this account – a little more from his since he earned more. Both of them had money left for personal spending.

Control

She had the overview over the current bills. She was not willing to let go of this responsibility, arguing that:

I don't want to leave that to someone else. I want to have control over the situation. I like that. I like to count money. Then there's never as much left as I think there will be. I am overly optimistic every time.

She made all decisions regarding savings, which implied that she suggested different forms of saving. They both had personal savings accounts, and she supervised the fairness in their savings, in other words, equal amount was saved every month by both partners.

Right to personal money

Both regarded it as important to have their own financial space. But they also regarded it as important to know about each other's spending for personal purposes, and could comment on this. The woman regarded herself as the big spender, she had a need to treat herself and be a bit reckless, but without a guilty conscience. The man was more future oriented and careful, wanting to save and collect. But he also had his financial space, and spent money on his own interests.

Ideal and practice

This couple reacted strongly against the vignette describing a couple in which the man had more to spend than the woman. Both partners were morally committed to joint finances, having always applied it themselves. He claimed: 'Separated economy is like preparing for divorce . . . we talk about *our* money, we never talk about hers or mine.' She claimed that having separate finances appeared to her as 'very strange . . . destructive'.

She reflected on the vignette about the use of the gift in terms of economic equality – the right of the fictitious woman to use the gift for herself depended on if there was a need to compensate a 'less privileged' party in the relationship. In other words, the use of the money gift was in her view conditional and dependent on a rightful allocation in the greater perspective. He was completely in favour of a joint use of the gift.

Summary

There were three couples in this category. They were all strongly in favour of the ideal that joint expenditure should take precedence over personal. In all couples, the women tended to have the main responsibility for expenditures and claimed to have a large influence over what was consumed. Both parties also supervised each other's personal consumption. In two of the couples, the economy was so meagre that the money overall covered only the joint expenses.

Joint economy as ideal but with elements of separate practice

Allocations

In this couple, there was no joint account for expenses, but there was a joint savings account that both parties made deposits into. His income paid for the rent, petrol and food – and hers for the rest.

Control

This couple represents an example where the woman claimed to have complete control over the finances, which meant that she was fully responsible for the family's budget. She administered the bills and had access to the husband's personal account, but he had no access to hers. Towards the end of every month, the couple went through the expenses, so in practice, he also had control. When it came to saving, the husband was in control – according to him, he was the one who would 'make sure it is done . . . otherwise it won't be done'. By controlling the saving, i.e. the amounts left over, he could also control the expenses in relation to the incomes.

The reasons as to why she took care of the economy were practical. She stated that he entrusted her with this task because of his overall trust in her. His view was that it was comfortable that she took care of everything. When he needed cash for himself, he asked her to set aside a sum for him. Thus, he did not want to be given money in the hand, which can be interpreted as symbolic of the fact that she does not give him money; she manages it and makes payments on request. He told the interviewer that she sometimes set aside less than the amount he had asked for. In this way, she was in charge of his financial space to a certain extent.

Right to personal money

The couple had created an economic division that would give each one of them equally sized financial scopes of action. The woman in this family perceived herself as having sufficient scope for personal consumption. In her view, equality is about fair distribution, and she controlled this distribution each month. Insight into the separate consumption would, however, be hidden from the other.

> Because I must admit . . . I think it's very important that you have that liberty that the other person does not know exactly everything you buy, but that you have a little to yourself. And of course, it's been pretty easy for me, since I've taken care of the economy.

Ideal and practice

Both argued with conviction that their finances should be seen as joint. The husband said: 'We put our money in a pile. We share everything and have as much for personal use.' In terms of the gift vignette, both claimed that it would be immoral that the person who received the gift would make an individual decision on its use. The wife declared:

> I would not have been able to make that journey. No, I don't think so. Because then I'd feel it would be wrong to him and the children. I would. Yes, disloyal, yes. Even if it'd be lovely I wouldn't do it, no.

She claimed that he would be angry if she would use the money on herself, and that she would use the money on her own only on condition that he agreed.

In terms of household consumption, their opinions were partially different, but they did not have conflicts regarding money. Rather, they had a power struggle, as both parties claimed individually.

Summary

This category was represented by eight couples. Characteristic of this model was that the joint economy had presidence over the personal, and that both parties should have equal amounts to spend for their own purposes. The women had the main responsibility for the budget, and made the decisions on the consumption. In the group, however, there were also several examples of men consuming more items than the women, or that they had a larger financial space.

Sharing and sense of justice

In all the couples studied, joint pooling was practised in one way or another, also in the couples where separate finances were regarded as an ideal to strive for. In fifteen out of twenty-two couples, a joint economy was regarded as an ideal. They claimed that they did not make any difference between 'yours' or 'mine', and that all the money was put in the same pot. Different kinds of joint ownership of capital assets, such as the house, were also a very common practice among the couples. However, the principle of joint ownership did not exclude some extent of practical division in ownership or savings. For instance, if one person received an inheritance, it was regarded as separate. Similarly, higher levels of contribution to the estate were also regarded as separate saving.

The majority of the couples thus applied some form of conscious agreement about how their incomes should be allocated to the joint or separate consumption. As we have seen, there are many variations of how fixed and day-to-day expenses are allocated in practice when it comes to organisation of the cash flow. In some cases, consultancy advice had been taken in order to work out a functioning model. This implied that allocations had been discussed in terms of justice and convenience. Several couples had joint accounts that both could make withdrawals from. Strikingly, none of them recognised any elements of injustice in their particular ways of organising the economy, even though the outcome in terms of personal consumption implied severe limitations for some of the women.

Among the patterns that we have discerned, different principles of justice form the basis for the togetherness created by the couple. In the first example, the principle was 'equal amount from each to the common good', regardless of income and personal debts. It was seen as fair that each partner should contribute the same amount and that the person who earned more should also keep more for personal needs. The implication of this principle in our examples was that the husband who earned more kept more. The kind of togetherness that this couple developed can be labelled 'market pricing' with reference to the typology developed by Fiske (1991, 1992). It is based on an individual orientation where the borders between you and me, yours and mine, are made clear. The unequal sharing was not regarded as unjust by the woman who had less money to dispose of, nor was it regarded as unjust by the man. She thought that their relationship was equal, since her ideal was to have control over her personal money. Personal autonomy was regarded as more important than equal sharing. In the other example, the same principle was applied, but the wife contributed her entire salary for joint consumption, and in addition, the husband had claimed the right to control all consumption, including hers. The outcome of this pattern was more or less the same as the first, that the husband had more financial freedom and spent more. The women had a guilty conscience when they purchased items for themselves. In the examples provided, this was not viewed as unfair, but both parties claimed that they lived in an equal relationship. To one woman, equality was strongly associated with controlling her *own* finances. To the other woman, the meaning of equality consisted of mutuality and a feeling of togetherness. Her husband gave her money, she perceived herself as a receiver of gifts, and that gave her a sense of dignity. In this couple, the partners had different ideals, but since the husband controlled the money, we can claim that the type of togetherness created was built on the principle of authority ranking with a needs-oriented justice as the legitimising principle.

The third pattern represented an economic togetherness that in Fiske's (1991, 1992) terminology would be referred to as communal sharing. The jointly shared was completely superior, and needs-oriented justice ruled. However, this category was not entirely pure. It was conditioned by low incomes that largely covered only that which was jointly shared. For a couple to have communal sharing as a superior principle could lead to conflicts in terms of separate consumption, or lead the couple to evolve into the fourth pattern.

The fourth category represented a combination of a fair allocation based on a needs-oriented ethic. The jointly shared pool was superior in principle, but just allocation was perceived as a prerequisite for realising the ideal. Just allocation meant equal amounts to each party, regardless of incomes. A very clear element in this category was that the women had the main responsibility for the economy, and were often in charge to a greater extent than the men. The economic togetherness created was what Fiske (1991, 1992) refers to as communal sharing but with a combination of needs-oriented justice and allocation according to the principle of equal amounts allocated from the surplus, if existing.

The results of the study provide a complex picture of the symbolic significance of joint and separate finances. Some couples referred to joint economy as an indication of the stability of the relationship. For instance, one woman said that she was protecting her personal finances in a much stricter way in the early phases of the partnership, when the economy was separate. Their moving towards a joint pooling was to her a confirmation of the stability and longevity of their relationship.

Among the studied couples, some argued with strong moral ardour that having a separate economy is equivalent to separation. The couples who advocated separate finances reacted equally strongly to the notion of having a joint economy. It was assumed that it would lead to a surveillance approach, that you had a hold on the other person and their consumption. Many emphasised the importance of having your own money to decide over, without the other person interfering in how it was spent. Even couples with separate economies, where one or both advocated the ideal, there was no strict division between yours and mine. Instead, a kind of fluid allocation was applied, where money was taken from either person without the connotation of lending. The important thing was the principle that each person should have their own money to decide over.

Having joint pooling as an economic principle was thus not regarded as equivalent to having an equal relationship per se. Joint economy could imply both increased economic freedom or diminished economic freedom, so that the personal consumption was subordinate in relation to the jointly shared. It is important to point out that the jointly shared does not have to be the equivalent with shared control or power over the allocation. Joint economy can coexist with both or only one party being in control over how the communal assets should be allocated.

In the households in our study, it was very common practice (eleven couples) that the women managed the money from the administration point of view. Among those who perceived themselves as having joint economies, it was frequently the women who managed the bills. In these cases, the woman could in some cases also be in control. However, where the man alone managed the finances, he also administered the bills in all cases. In a majority of these cases, the husband had a significantly higher salary than his wife.

Control over joint and separate money

Some of the couples had previously amalgamated their finances, but later transferred to separate accounts. The reason for this was difficulties with cash flow control, and no money being left over for saving purposes. One party may have been perceived as the bigger spender, and the other as more parsimonious. Different views on money led to conflicts. By separating the accounts, the couples achieved both overview and practical control. As shown in the previous section, ways of organising the flow were significant in terms of personal freedom to consume: if all incomes are placed in a joint pool, it becomes very relevant if one or both control that joint pool. The control is thus related to decision-making regarding household money and freedom in terms of personal consumption, i.e. the right to personal money. This is linked to how money is viewed, and how these different perceptions are handled.

In this section, we intend to go deeper into family dynamics by presenting various perceptions of how money should be used. How did the couples make decisions regarding money allocated to the joint household? How did they make decisions on personal consumption? It was not uncommon that different perceptions prevailed regarding the use of money, what purchases should be made, what purposes one should save for and the amounts involved. This could be handled in different ways, and the differences in perception were not necessarily regarded as conflicts. In this study, there were only a few (six women and four men) who claimed that they had explicit conflicts about money. How common is this? In the study from 1992, the following question was asked: 'Does it happen that issues regarding the use of your incomes lead to conflicts between you and your partner?' Almost 50 per cent of the women and 42 per cent of the men replied that they sometimes had such conflicts, but only 4 per cent of both genders replied that they had such conflicts often. Slightly more than half of both genders thus replied that they never had conflicts about money. However, this should not be interpreted in terms of an absence of different perceptions regarding the actual use of the money. Conflicts about money are usually quite loaded, since they touch upon several dimensions in togetherness – the need for personal freedom and consideration for the needs of others, perceptions of justice and merit. Money is a taboo subject, and is not normally discussed openly with others. Simultaneously, it is well known that money or the 'gap between resource and need' is a recurring source of differences in opinions in families (Lennéer-Axelsson and Thylefors 1996). Since money has a deep symbolic value in togetherness, it can be hypothesised that various strategies are created for the management of different perceptions about how the money should be used with the purpose of avoiding conflict. We will present a few examples of such strategies.

Two main groups were discerned in our sample – a group in which both partners claimed that the woman was restrictive and the man was more indulgent, and a group in which both claimed that the man was more restrictive and the woman more indulgent. It is interesting to note that both parties, independently of each other, presented a similar view of the economic dynamics in the couple relationship.

Restrictive woman, indulgent man

The first group represented most couples in the sample. The group included all the (four) couples where the women earned more than their husbands. Remarkably, the men in this group claimed to be rather uninterested in consumption, or they claimed that the consumption that was interesting to them could be identified as shared.

In all cases apart from two, the women in this group applied a strategy for creating financial scope aimed at decision-making or at least having control over the economy in the family. This was done by saving money, which was mainly personal, and through the development of rational consumer behaviour. Purchases were meticulously planned, whether they were personal, such as buying clothes for the family (sometimes including the husband), or made for the household. In order to save money, they restricted their personal consumption. The issue at stake was principally the desire to be in control and make decisions regarding purchases for the home and the children, but not so much in relation to themselves. The men appreciated the women's consumer competence, and claimed that the whole family benefited.

One common strategy was to save money in a personal account that was used for joint expenses and in another account for the children, where e.g. the child allowances were deposited. If discussions arose regarding the purchases, the women stated that they covered the costs themselves, and in that way there was no need for discussions. Having personal money meant that conflicts could be avoided. It was also conspicuous that in many cases, the women saved money given to them by their own parents.

In one couple, the woman claimed that she was the one who planned the economy and instigated changes – she had a long-term economic view when it came to the welfare of the family. She wanted to be one step ahead. The man did not share this view. When money was accessible, he wanted to spend it, without much thought as to how or why it disappeared. In another couple, the woman said that both of them could end up with a couple of hundred pounds left over from their salaries:

> Well, then I am wise and keep it in the bank, and he, well I have no idea where it goes, I don't even care to look, but he is never left with a few hundred, it gets spent along the way. But I have always saved, so I have something like . . . well, roughly £5000 in my account, but he has nothing.

She regarded this money, which sometimes had amounted to a few thousand, not as hers but earmarked for joint expenses:

> I gladly use it for the family, but it feels good to have it in my account, for example when I want to go on a mini-break, I can withdraw them just like

that. But I wouldn't mind paying for some armchairs that I want. But I can't do that as long as he is totally against it.

The latter part of the quote is characteristic of the women who saved in order to create financial scope of action. Joint purchases were rarely made without agreement. The road to agreement could be long and lined with nagging. The women claimed to use wearing-down tactics to enforce their will, because they knew that sooner or later, they would reach their goals.

The overall impression of the interviews with the couples in this group was that they rather consciously applied an equal balancing of incomes and day-to-day expenses. Disputes regarding money did occur, but seldom flared up into conflicts. Few of these couples regarded themselves as financially unequal.

Restrictive man, indulgent woman

The second group consisted of couples where the conditions were reversed – he wanted to restrain and restrict, she wanted to spend. Characteristic of this couple was that the man earned significantly more than the woman. It was also the husband who handled the economy and managed the bills. In these families, the wife wanted to spend more than the husband for *joint* purposes. It could be interior decoration, travels or consumption for the children. A recurring theme was that both claimed that the wife spent very little on herself. She was restrictive in that regard, since she had little money of her own and was not keen on asking for money for personal expenses. However, the husband spent money on himself without hesitation. Her low personal consumption was thus caused by other factors than the limited personal consumption in the first group, in which a low level of consumption aimed at creating an economic buffer zone and control.

In terms of objective measures based on the criteria of sameness, these families were economically unequal since the men earned more money, had financial control and contributed significantly more to the communally shared pool. The women also paid for joint expenses according to models that left them with very little left over for personal expenses. Despite this, all women and men in this group perceived themselves as economically equal. The women claimed to have the same economic living standards as the men, and often owned half of the property – a significant symbolic issue, in addition to the actual economic importance of ownership.

In terms of decisions regarding joint consumption, the women had to create strategies aimed at making the men agree with their wishes, since they were dependent on the husband's will to spend. One wife described a situation of choice between two items, where she suggested the slightly cheaper and simpler item to the husband first. He asked her if she did not think that the slightly more expensive item was better. 'Sure I think so. But I didn't tell him. Sometimes it's fun and games.'

Women's stories about strategies for making the men agree to larger purchases were in fact similar to the ones described by the women with money, namely nagging, coaxing, persuasion and arguments. Those stories were rarely told by the men in our material. However, this does not imply that the men did not have to convince and argue for the larger purchases.

The woman in the quote above had a slightly guilty conscience because she contributed only a little money. This in turn affected her ability to use money for her own needs. The husband himself was restrictive, which enhanced her urge to restrain. In order to resolve this conflict, she wanted to start working more in order to earn more money for the household. Although they both claimed that there were no conflicts about money, the woman made the following statement:

> We don't disagree with each other, I can't say that, but we damn well talk about money. Because I can come along and ask 'Can I buy this', he thinks, 'Do you have to', but we don't fight. I get the feeling that I have to find out if we have money so that I can go and buy my thing. Because I don't really know. If it's something big, something more expensive . . . Well, I still don't buy . . . but according to my husband, I'm a trigger-happy spender because he's not at all like that. And then you become trigger-happy in comparison, but compared to acquaintances and girlfriends, I'm not at all. He sees me that way but that's typical men.

Another woman communicated a similar story, but in her case the element of conflict was significantly greater, according to descriptions provided by both parties. She claimed that her husband could get irritated with her if she had spent more money than was planned. The husband's strategy was to plan larger purchases, and he wanted to make the decisions. He acknowledged that he sometimes said: 'I earn more and we'll have to adjust to that', i.e. he made the decisions about what and when to buy. At the same time, he claimed that he could outweigh his consumption against his work, where he was given a lot in terms of dinners and travelling. Against that background, he meant that he could treat her to her own purchases. He did not think it was necessary for him to discuss larger purchases – if he felt that something was needed, he bought it.

It was common for these couples to refer to their own and each other's conditions of upbringing in order to explain why their views on money were different. Financial scarcity during childhood in these stories often account for both urges to spend and restrain. Explanations based on childhood, and not on their differences in individual, financial conditions, were used to legitimise the other person's controlling approach.

The role of close kin in economic negotiations

In conversations with the couples it emerged that parents have acted as a buffer during different phases of the couple's life, both economically and socially. Slightly more women (twelve women and nine men) had received economic support from a parent. Many women had been given financial backing in a personal form, i.e. the money was earmarked for her and was aimed at providing her with a buffer to manage economic crises or to add some luxury in her everyday life. It could also be in the form of aid to purchase a house or apartment. In the case of house purchases, the money was often given as a loan, which later became a gift.

It does not appear as though the parents' support contributed to the women becoming more indulgent, since the restrictive women were the ones who had received most support. In the men's case, it was predominantly the indulgent men who had received support. Based on the limited material available in this study, it is not possible to make assumptions about how representative this pattern is.

The women were positive to the support they had received, and claimed that it contributed to a sense of independence. For instance, one woman claimed that through her parents' support, she felt as though she could continue on her own if something should happen in her relationship.

> But of course, if you start nibbling at it, it will finish. It's not as if you'd take off, but it's a security to maybe be able to buy a flat somewhere. I don't have enough money to buy without a mortgage but I have a basis. So I am in a different position compared to many other women ... it's incredibly important. Even if I never think about it and never use it ... it's there for me if something should happen. You don't know anything about life tomorrow, you only know about what you're living now.

Portraying oneself as financially self-sufficient to their parents was very important to both parties, and was especially emphasised in the interviews. However, for the women it was rarely associated with ambivalence to turn to their parents. The men were more restrictive in turning to their parents for help in a financial crisis. They preferred to borrow money and repay swiftly, to show that they were economically independent. In some cases, the men expressed ambivalence in relation to the economic support given to their wives, despite the fact that it benefited the household.

Different understandings of equality in allocation of money

What conclusions can be drawn from these results concerning the implications for economic equality? There is no unambiguous answer, since the picture of various set-ups is complex, and the criteria for what is equal vary. Taking into account how both men and women perceive justice in their set-ups, we can conclude that both the men and the women in the couples perceived themselves as being economically equal. This perception was based on that they perceived themselves to be living on similar economic standards and that financial decisions were handled relatively free from conflicts, i.e. there was agreement and decisions were not railroaded. Only two men and two women regarded themselves as economically unequal. The two men argued that they earned more and spent more, thus did not have the same economic standard of living as their wives. In both cases, the couples had relatively separate finances. One of the women (not in these two couples) argued that she was in an unequal relationship, because she could not buy what she wanted without her husband protesting. The husband, on the other hand, could pursue his interests with the child. The other woman felt unequal because she could not contribute as much to the household as her husband. Her lesser contribution was combined with the fact that her husband was uninterested in consumption, and she felt obliged to ask about and discuss the purchases that she wanted to make. This made her feel dependent on him.

Judging equality with the eyes of the observer, it can be concluded that in most families, the men had greater economic power than the women through their higher earning and higher levels of contribution to the communally shared pool. Due to their higher earnings, the partners perceived that the men had a self-evident role in the decision-making of the household and the personal consumption. As a consequence the men did not feel obliged to anchor their economic decisions to the extent that women did. This situation resulted in economic insecurity among the women regarding their scope of action in terms of their own consumption. The interviews showed that for women, joint consumption was given priority over personal consumption to a higher extent than for the men, thereby restricting women's personal consumption. Similar results appeared in the study by Nyman (2002), who writes about an economic 'grey zone' which is not part of the allocation agreements – day-to-day expenditures that are involved in the types of responsibilities that women often represent (for instance buying gifts for friends and children's parties).

We have noted a female strategy to gain control in order to establish a better bargaining position. This strategy implied saving and suppressing the personal consumption in order to gain a larger control over the joint expenditures. The women also gained economic power through taking initiatives for the joint consumption process. A part of this strategy consisted of convincing, wearing down and nagging through a decision-making process that was to be perceived as joint. This democratic decision-making strategy was an important factor in managing the men's greater economic scope of action. Through this, the women compensated for their lower incomes. Similar strategies were used by women who earned slightly more than or as much as their husbands.

So what is economic equality in couple relationships? A pure joint economy is one possible criterion. Another consists of equal division and agreement. Being in control and making joint decisions regarding consumption is yet another criterion. We have been able to separate four patterns of economic management in the couples, based on perceptions of what is morally right and the practice developed in everyday life for allocation and control of the economy. We want to emphasise that both strictly separate economies and fully joint economies were conciliatory with different types of control. In both types of economy, there are examples of male control and dominance of the economy. Both forms were shown to imply differing economic standards in the couple relationship. Since joint economy was combined with separate economy, both parties were often in control, although the women most often handled it in practice.

Our interpretation of equality derived from the couple's own judgement is that it is relative to a combination of criteria. It is both a matter of what is experienced as fair allocation of money, and what is represented by togetherness in terms of money and consumption. The allocation per se carries symbolic importance. Even if the allocation does not lead to complete sameness in resources, they have been subject to discussion and found to represent a fair allocation within the relationship framework. This gives weight to the impression that the economy implies equality. It is the procedure rather than the outcomes that make the allocation appear as fair. This is an aspect of relational ethics that has been demonstrated in studies on perceptions of justice (Kellerhals et al. 1997). That the women in certain couples make more payments, or rather, end up with less money for themselves, is connected to the division of labour in the household. The division gives them a greater responsibility for the joint household, and thus also the joint consumption.

Posing boundaries and managing conflicts

In previous chapters, we have described how men and women in couple relationships divide household labour between each other, and what their reasoning regarding this issue is. Furthermore, we have presented the models developed by these couples to allocate money and property, saving and consumption. In this chapter, we will take a closer look at communicative strategies used when managing conflicts and opposing interests in negotiations regarding allocation. We will reconnect with the theoretical review in Chapter 4, using concepts to describe negotiations, conflict resolution, power and influence in interpersonal relationships. What may be perceived as a conflict varies both within and between couples. It is not uncommon that conflicts are perceived as pure confrontation, which carries a negative connotation.[1] In Chapter 4, we described conflict as a process in which differences in interests, resources or aims are handled. We ascribe to the term 'conflict' its wider definition. Our aim is to describe how couples handle opposing interests in decision-making that concern both great and small issues in everyday life. The basis of the analysis is constituted by the couples' stories about decision-making and what situations have led to conflicts. The couples in the interview situation were asked to describe situations that they come to think of spontaneously, and provide concrete examples of situations that have given rise to differences in perceptions. We used vignettes in order to make common everyday dilemmas more concrete. We also asked the interviewees straight out how they perceive their influence on how decisions are made in the family and who usually gets the last word. Furthermore, we asked how they perceive the division of influence in different areas – if they think one of them is in charge to a greater or lesser extent, e.g. regarding decisions with financial implications. We have also asked them to describe who takes the initiative for purchases, and how such decisions were made.

A particular aspect in the management of conflicts and disagreements is how the individual poses boundaries between the self and the other in the relationship. Negotiating for your personal time is also a form of boundary creation – a way of obtaining self-governance. This is also a theme treated in this section, mediated by the question if one actually has any personal time.

We also asked the couples questions about their relationships with the children, their views on child-rearing, whether there is agreement or conflicts in issues regarding the children. Our interest for equality and negotiations in couple relationships places the main focus on how parents handle different opinions concerning the children. The couples' different parenting and conflict management styles are thus the focus of the analysis, rather than the relationship between parents and children.

Conflicts in numbers

In the conversations with the couples, it emerged that differences mainly concern the division of labour in the home, relationships with the children, consumption and the access to personal time. How common is it that these types of issues lead to conflicts?

In the 1992 study, the couples were asked if they had conflicts regarding the home and the children. Of all respondents, 24 per cent of the women and 18 per cent of the men claimed to have conflicts in the home.[2] Four conflict areas were studied – household labour, money, childcare and attitudes to child-rearing. The most common source of conflict was money: 50 per cent of women and 42 per cent of the men claimed to have conflicts regarding the use of their incomes. As mentioned previously, 35 per cent of the women and 25 per cent of the men claimed to have conflicts regarding household work at least once a week. The differences between the genders were particularly strong among couples in the upper socio-economic strata. A comparison shows that 54 per cent of the women in upper-level professions and 28 per cent of the men on the same level claimed to have conflicts regarding household chores.

Women's experiences of conflicts in the home correlated with time spent at work – full-time workers and women in higher-level professions experienced higher levels of conflicts than the men in similar conditions. Furthermore, experiences of household work as being heavy were also associated with conflicts in the home. These correlations were similar for both genders. Additionally, having more children was associated with more conflicts, with the women also experiencing more conflicts than the men.

Children as a source of conflict

In the 1992 study, working with the children was experienced as conflict-laden by 20 per cent of both genders. On questions about child-rearing being experienced as conflict-laden, a slightly smaller proportion of both genders (approximately 14 per cent) replied in the positive. The differences in the replies can be explained by agreement between the parties on a general level of approach, but different styles being applied in practice when controlling the children. The issues were e.g. homework, table manners, cleaning and tidying, punctuality, clothing purchases, having friends over, activities etc. Applying control in such matters was perceived as work with children.

The different ways of interacting with the children were investigated in the study by asking the participants to compare themselves with their partners as parents. The results showed for example that slightly more than 40 per cent of the women and 33 per cent of the men claimed to have a different view of child-rearing than their partner/spouse, while 43 per cent of the men expressed the opinion that the women were better with the children than they were. More women (29 per cent) than men (18 per cent) considered their partner to be more impatient. A greater share of the women (31 per cent) than the men (8 per cent) thought that their partner spent too little time with the children. The results show that the couples were different in their approach to the children, and that in many cases, these differences were associated with conflict.

An overwhelming majority of the interviewed couples in the in-depth study claimed to agree on their fundamental ideas about what the children needed to learn and how they should behave in the family and in the community. On the other hand, several couples mentioned that the children were a source of repeated conflict or opposing viewpoints. It was predominantly the women who claimed that the children created conflicts between the spouses. One type of conflict was based on the women's experience of a lack of their husband's engagement when it came to the day-to-day lives of their children. Another type consisted of a perceived inability to pose boundaries in relation to the children; yet another one was related to a difference in style when it came to the children. These three types of conflicts are associated with the women having the main responsibility for the children, and thereby having a more active role in balancing the children's, the husband's and their own needs. We will illustrate these types of child-related problems with a few examples.

One woman described many conflicts, many frustrations and strong wills concerning herself and the children: 'Having children is heavy. I don't think I'm made for it. I'm not that kind of a mother.' To her, 'that kind of a mother' represents a person who puts her own interest in the background, and the needs of the children and the family in the foreground. Many conflicts stemmed from the perception that she did not give the children enough positive content. 'It's mostly tough,' she stated. 'I think they wear me down and their fighting with each other also wears a lot, I think.' She viewed it as conflictual that she as an adult had to show respect for the children and be considerate, while she thought they were not respectful, 'they have no respect whatsoever.'

One man, who had chosen a passive stance in relation to the children, claimed that he did not have much to contribute. He justified his own passivity by saying that his wife had always been active and engaged, 'so it's become very natural in our family that she takes care of everything.' On the other hand, he could have opinions on the conduct of the children. Both partners in this couple claimed that they had different views on how the children should behave during meals, cleaning of their rooms and doing school work. She said:

> When they eat, he always goes: 'When I was a child, you finished everything on the plate' and I don't like that. OK, let them have a taste, but if they don't like it, they don't like it.

She did not think this was an issue to bring up with the children; you have to respect the children's feelings. She had ambitions to teach them how to save, think forward, not to spend impulsively and make demands for them to do household chores. She tried to push these issues forward, but was unable to persevere in the end. She presented herself as the more benevolent parent, or in other words, the one who could not resist their unwillingness to comply, apart from on certain occasions. She did not perceive the differences in opinion with her husband as a conflict issue. This was due to the fact that she had the greater say. In her opinion, the person who spends the most time at home will not have the energy to nag. On the other hand, she claimed that it is important to explain to the children where the differences between the parents' opinions lie.

In one couple, the woman said: 'He is very determined when it comes to child-rearing and I think it's good for them.' At the same time, she claimed: 'Yes, and then I think it's important that I am the softer one, I mitigate things a little.' She thought that he scared the children to obedience, and tried to make him soften his approach. Discussions about this issue did not occur in front of the children, but after they had gone to bed. The husband described himself as a dominating person, but did not perceive himself as scary. Dominance to him was more of a clear and exact posing of boundaries, i.e. by roaring or ramming his fist on the table. He claimed that she also thought it was OK to ram the fist on the table. She, on the other hand, claimed that he got angry when she brought the issue to discussion and tried to influence him. 'He is very stubborn and finds it difficult to take in my opinion.' She tried to mitigate the effects of his rough ways on the children by talking to them. To herself, she explained that it was important to have rules, and in principle, she agreed with him and the rules that he applied. She also gave credit to his engagement in the family and the children that he wanted to rear them into engaging in sensible leisure activities in their free time, as well as to the fact that he wanted them to be together and consume practical and useful things. She was more dedicated to glamour, not only for herself but also for the children. However, she felt forced to be part of what he wanted. In order to show him and herself that she also thought of good child rearing, she attempted to do things with them in her free time, although she was tired. However, the children also preferred to stay at home and do nothing. The ambivalence in her approach was particularly clear in her emphasis of 'not being self-eradicating in any way. But there is so much on when you have children. More and more, you think less about yourself.' She thus chose to be the way she thought a good mother or parent should be, but simultaneously experienced a conflict between his view and how she herself wanted to be as a mother and a person. This conflict situation clearly highlights the tension between authenticity and self-governance/sacrifice that was discussed in Chapter 4.

Controlling the children with rules or arguments

These descriptions and quotes illustrate common types of differences regarding the children in the couples studied. Almost half of the couples expressed that they had differences in opinions when it came to how they controlled the children, how they tried to influence them or pose behavioural boundaries. The differences followed a traditional gender pattern – the father often imposed clear boundaries, used a sharp tone, gave clear directions about boundaries and was principled. The mother coaxed and gave in, imposed less clear boundaries and let the situation determine how hard she would push her convictions. The day-to-day situations that were mentioned were mainly bedtimes, food, meals and consumption.

Many couples claimed that they tried to avoid confronting each other's convictions in front of the children – perhaps to steer clear of overt fighting in their presence. That their convictions differed was still clear to the children, however. The different styles were a significant cause of conflict between the parents, and gave rise to discussion and quarrels.

Expressions of these gender-typical styles varied, and reflected different values. The mother's style was referred to as lax or nagging, both by the man and the woman. This implies that mothers are inconsequential that they admonish too weakly and mildly, which can be perceived as negative. It can also imply that mothers have a softer style, whereas fathers are tougher. The reverse case also occurred – that the mothers were described as tougher, and the fathers as more psychological and negotiating, calm and reasoning. However, it is interesting to note that none of the men was described as lax or inconsequential, and the women were not described as psychological and negotiating. Many men claimed that their wife had the final word and decided over the children. That is, the fathers passed the responsibility to the mothers for small and big issues in the children's detailed, day-to-day practical care and rearing. None of the participants referred to the men as being passive or lax in this context.

Thus we can conclude that there is a clear gender dimension in how the couples perceived their different styles, and that these were given particular labels in the narratives. For the women, being soft – i.e. open for negotiations, listening and being prone to adapt according to the children's arguments – was perceived as female and wrong. If men behaved in a similar fashion, by first coming on too strongly, then getting a guilty conscience and apologising, there were no negative connotations, since the apology was interpreted as recognition that the tactic was wrong. In principle, all participants claimed that their own style was the right one. Different methods were used to either accept the other's style or avoid direct confrontation and criticism in front of the children. Some of them took to fighting immediately, and had overt quarrels about who was right or wrong. This was particularly the case for women who had greater influence in the family, and in those cases where the men governed. They were less prepared to change and try to adapt to the men. For example, one woman was described as significantly more permissive than the man. This caused endless conflicts between them. She knew that he thought she was too lax, but there were no signs of her agreement with this opinion. She made most household decisions and was fully responsible for everything, including child-rearing, with the exception of those instances when she was not at home – in those cases, the husband took care of things his way. Another woman had the opinion that her and her husband's different styles complemented each other, but she was in charge most of the time. Women who expressed such an approach claimed that their styles were more effective, less counter-productive and more respectful.

Among women who presented themselves as more dominant, there was a certain ambivalence associated with their own style. They took in their husbands' criticism of them, claiming to know that they were doing wrong. One woman claimed, for instance, that the man was too harsh and scared the children to obedience. At the same time, she also thought it was good that he was determined and that she should also be like him, or rather, like one should be. On the other hand, she thought it was positive that she occupied the mild role, smoothing things over, comforting and calming the children. She was thus not prepared to change her style, but thought that he was right and that his style was necessary. In practice, this could imply that she was silent and let the man carry on, but changed his orders when he had left. It could also imply that they tried to avoid potentially confrontational situations, by going off on her own to buy clothes for the children in order not to end up in discussions about prices, sizes and models.

One reason why the women persevered in their styles was that they spent more time with the children, knew them better and were aware of how best to control them. Reversibly, just by spending a lot of time with the children could mean that they did not have the energy to put up a fight and have conflicts with the children. According to one woman, the reason for her lax discipline was that she was as sensitive as a person. She disliked spats and got a guilty conscience when she was harsh with the children:

> I am so sensitive that I think I let go too much. I don't like fighting with the children or about the children. I get such a guilty conscience when I yell at them.

She also thought that she was the one who treated the children unfairly most often: one of them received more attention than the other. When asked who got the last word in issues concerning the children, she said that she did not know, but that she often chose to be quiet and walk away:

> I don't know who gets the last word, but I feel as if 'No, I can't fight any more, I'd rather be silent' and then I walk away. I don't like fighting. I shut off. It's probably been more that way the last years, no I can't do it.

At the same time, she maintained that she was not the one who remained quiet too often – her husband was.

> No, I think I'm the one who nags and carries on very much and he says nothing. And then I get mad because he doesn't say anything, he is calmer. And when he sometimes really lets things out, I almost get scared and wonder 'What now?' Then the issue is really something for him to get angry. Then he has kind of had enough. I am more of a 'bark not bite' kind of person.

We also noticed gender differences in terms of language style. Saying it like it is, putting your foot down without an invitation to discussion, was perceived as harsher, whereas looking the other way was perceived as soft and not so good. It was perceived as a lax and a less desirable approach. The person who was prepared to look the other way, break rules and adapt the rule to the situation was perceived as inconsequential, viewed from a justice perspective. From the relational ethics perspective, this meant being perceptive, being prepared to listen to the other party's argument (in this case, the child's) and being prepared to negotiate. Several women in our material perceived the relationship ethics approach as negative, that is, the style that was not the officially correct style. You have to be principled and rule-oriented. But at the same time, they argued that the relational ethics style felt right for them, and that they stuck to it when the husband was not present (if he adhered to the justice-oriented principle). When conflicts arose concerning these different styles, many women felt that they could not manage to assert themselves and their opinion relative to that of their partner. This led to increased insecurity in their demeanour, since they were aware that they were acting incorrectly. On the other hand, they maintained their style in practice, of which there were several examples in our study.

Time for self

Freedom was an important dimension in the discussion about equality and division of labour in the home. It was mainly the women who articulated the need for freedom. This theme was more or less absent in the men's narratives – they hardly spoke about freedom at all. Some men mentioned that they had their need for freedom satisfied through work. In this context, freedom was attributed a special meaning that was associated with the possibility to develop as an individual through work. Men with creative professions in particular spoke about freedom in this sense when asked whether they had time to themselves as individuals. Freedom did thus not imply leisure time. The women related to freedom in terms of an intensive desire or in terms of something they had actively given up for the children and the family. Most women, however, expressed a strong need for time to themselves. Some referred to this time as 'holy time'.

One woman said:

> I want to get out all the time. Go travelling or do something else, just leave home . . . I have a great need for getting away from here . . . I sometimes long for that feeling of freedom.

This woman claimed that she was being 'suffocated' by duties at home and at work. It was mainly the household work, but also the children that she experienced as suffocating. Several women meant that their choice to work part time was associated with the need to gain freedom, time to care for themselves. The woman above was an example of this. She had chosen to work part time in order to take care of herself, but still did not consider her free time to be very free. She considered herself as equal in relation to her husband, but freedom was more important than equality to her.

To one of the women, the lack of personal time was one of her biggest problems. Her experience was that she had far too little time on her own. This concerned several, small needs, she claimed – doing things on a whim, having a bath, going out to eat: 'No, every time I feel like I have to do that [set her needs aside] I am angry, mad, in general pretty angry.' The strategies she had developed to care for herself were connected with the household – by choosing to do the shopping, she got away from the house and was able to stroll around and window shop while she did the food shopping. Looking for bargains was her interest, it was pleasurable to her. Another strategy was to do huge quantities of laundry, which required her presence in the communal laundry utility room. In there, she could sit down and read a book.

One woman said:

> It has always been the case in our family that you should be able to do something once a week. That's the minimum. Last year, I had one night a week. And it is completely natural for both of us that we give it to each other, I think so. Free time must be divided just like the economy and household work. It is important that the right to free time is not questioned.

Another woman claimed that she needed to be alone in order to find inner strength: 'As a woman, I have to charge my batteries by being alone sometimes.' She sometimes chose solitude consciously, unplugging the telephone and listening to music. She perceived having time at her disposal and getting in touch with herself as a condition for survival. To her, Friday was her time off, and she regarded it as her own time. She met up with her girlfriends who also had Fridays off. She could potter about in the kitchen and read the newspaper – be free. She referred to having abstained from a course (that she had taken previously and enjoyed very much) because it would have implied a lock-up of time. 'Then I won't get pleasure from it. That way, everything has to be done by the Thursday.' Work was the factor that made her unwilling to commit further.

One woman considered free time as having a central value, which could be found in a relationship only if both had these values and provided room for it to be realised in practice. To this woman, freedom was consequently a central element of togetherness, almost a prerequisite. According to her, the issue was generosity, being able to grant this to one another.

The women did not describe themselves as lacking freedom because their husbands were restricting them, i.e. openly stopping them from being themselves. The issue was not having time to meet others or engage in personal interests. It was rather the feeling of duty and demand, of others being dependent on their presence and engagement, that created the need for free time. Freedom was thus viewed in terms of being free from duties – whether they stemmed from work or home. Free time could be used at work, however – for professional development and education. But it had to be a free choice, associated with pleasure and engagement, not something that would legitimise the room for free time.

How did the women gain time for themselves? A common way of achieving this was to work part time. Women who had chosen this strategy, e.g. having one free day per week, had done so in order to care for themselves. The principal motivation was thus not keeping up with the household work. On the contrary, household work was what stood in the way of the freedom that the women wanted. Therefore, they were faced by a dilemma when they chose to work part time, since the time off work was regarded by both themselves and their surrounding as time freed for household work.

Another strategy was to piece together times that suited everybody. Many women claimed that the personal time had to be adapted to the family or the men. They chose times that did not coincide with that of the others – odd time, early mornings or late nights. One woman said:

> But it's better than choosing times that collide with my husband's work hours, for example, because it only causes irritation. He gets home too late and I get too late for my thing, and the whole thing falls apart. So now I think it works great, I think I can do lots of stuff on my own.

As was shown in one of the above examples, one strategy could be to weave the time to yourself into the household work, by choosing tasks that meant getting away, e.g. on shopping trips or spending time in the communal laundry room.

It can be hard to gain acceptance for the need for free time. The women felt that such time must be legitimised by a particular activity, or be taken from blocks of time that did not coincide with the needs and interests of others. It was borrowed time. One man referred to his wife's strong demands for time to herself in terms of hope that she would be able to tie it to work, like he did. 'I have made sure that much of that is part of my work . . . I get incredibly absorbed and it enriches me. It is my own time.' By tying it to his work, he gained a greater legitimacy for his need than her, since her need for time to herself was not so much connected to work, but to personal control.

For the women, the need for free time is explicitly associated with the need to pose boundaries for the self. In so doing, they run risks of encountering disagreements and conflicts. This is an important element of the whole theme of division of labour in the home. It is expressed as an inner conflict, as a tension between normative duties and the ability to free oneself of them – a struggle between duty and authenticity, following your own needs. The boundaries of the self also constitute an important part of the labour in creating togetherness, and touch the central theme of reconciling individuation and togetherness. Care and relationship work do not arise spontaneously in discussions regarding the division of labour in the household – it is weaved into the work itself and in planning all that is daily life. We interpret the words said about freedom not only as an expression of a struggle to gain relief in this work, but also as a struggle to free oneself of the ruling gender norms.

Different styles of conflict resolution

In previous chapters, we have given detailed presentations of types of governance for the division of household labour. One type consisted of governance by one party or attempts by one party to direct the division of labour in line with his or her own expectations. The second type consisted of joint governance or a lack of governance in practice. In each category, we have been able to discern several variations. In seven couples, the woman steered towards an equal division of labour of some kind. In five couples, both parties steered towards a traditional division of labour, and in two cases, the woman steered towards the same.

The source of conflict that permeated throughout the analysis of governance in all couples was the issue of norms or criteria for good enough housekeeping. It was mainly the women who imposed norms, and the men resisted them, although some of them were prepared to make concessions. In some couples, there was no such resistance, since they both cooperated. Taking part in the household work was seen by these men as an important factor in terms of their autonomy.

In the narratives, we have seen several examples of how women failed in their negotiations aimed at increasing the participation of the men. The question is why some have achieved a better division of labour based on their point of view, while the majority of those who wanted change have not been particularly successful. We shall now scrutinise the strategies of men and women in conflict resolution regarding the division of labour.

In our analysis of how couples handle their differences, we aim to identify strategies of conflict management in terms of the models presented in Chapter 4. The first model described the individual's perceptions of the self and of the interests and needs of others (see Figure 1, p. 32). The second model describes different types of conflict strategies that result from how the parties pursue their conflicting interests in relation to one another (Figure 2 , p. 35).

Couples with competing strategies

In this section, we shall describe two couples who in our opinion apply competing strategies of conflict resolution. In both couples, the wives earned more than their husbands. Formally, the women occupied positions on a higher-level status compared to their men. The impact of the formal levels of status within these couples cannot be evaluated in these examples; we can but conclude that the women in these two cases had economic power. This power had been strengthened by the women's initiative in taking control of the joint household finances, and by their creation of economic buffers for themselves and the jointly shared pool. The buffer was a result of economising and savings, and it provided scope for making several costly decisions – holiday plans, purchases for the home and for the children, and personal consumption. (These types of economic strategies are described in Chapter 7.) The economic strategies were laborious but also provided scope for competing strategies when it came to conflicts. The men in both of these families claimed to be uninterested in money and in interfering with the day-to-day financial decision-making. In addition, they saw themselves as having a personal financial scope of action that sufficed for their needs. Both women described themselves as governing in the family. They had the ambition to negotiate agreements regarding the division of labour. In both cases, the partners had very different views on the reality of their division of labour – overall, the men claimed that it was equal, and the women did not. This made it difficult for either of them to make concessions.

Levels of conflict in these couples were judged as high by themselves, which also led to high levels of frustration. In her description of their conflicts, one of the women said: 'Everything is said straight out; all issues come out in the open. Nothing is hidden.' Her husband confirmed this picture: 'We are both blood and fire, very direct towards one another but also very generous.' This was an intensity that displayed not only criticism but also generosity and praise. She explained:

> We get extremely angry but he always takes the initiative to ask for forgiveness. For him it is much easier to do so than for me. I sulk until he asks for forgiveness. I don't know why, but it has always been like this.

In the second couple, an intensive tempo and a high level of conflicts was also described. The woman in this couple was in a very conflict-laden situation – her perspective of self and others was strongly imprinted by role regulations, duties and musts. These factors created forced situations for both her and the other family members, which in turn led to a high intensity of conflicts.

In both cases, the women expressed high standards of what is important in family care, what is acceptable for tasks such as cleaning and childcare. In both couples, the women appear to be trapped in a model of internalised, normative rules. In relation to the model presented in Chapter 4, which described different perspectives of the self and others, we can interpret their situation as being high in family influence, but circumscribed by an unselfish approach – which means that they presented themselves as being ruled by the terms and conditions of others. This is reinforced by their presentation of themselves as governed by the conditions of others. The men in these couples did not perceive themselves as governed by general duties, nor did they see themselves as governing, but rather as governed by their wives, who actively wished for them to accept their norms. These norms were not subject to negotiation, since the men perceived them as being tied to the women's personalities.

In one couple, the husband referred to fundamental differences between himself and his wife. By labelling the differences as fundamental, they perceived fighting as being pointless. Both stuck stubbornly to their views, which led to confrontation of emotions. His concessions in these conflicts occurred because he was quick to forgive and resolve things emotionally. By avoiding his counter-strategies, she let herself be governed by the demands she perceived as necessary to live up to. This was not a matter of conflict resolution, but rather conflict diffusion for the sake of maintaining the relationship.

In the other couple, the woman's wish for more time to herself was a recurring cause of conflicts regarding the division of labour. He claimed that her frustration over lack of time was not connected to him, but to an inner conflict in her:

> I feel as though I have very little guilt in this, even if I have had to take the blame many times. In my opinion, I have been the one to say: go ahead, absolutely, I completely understand you. Take a week in a spa or whatever you want if you feel it's your thing.

In his own interpretation, he made it into a gender issue:

> I don't know if it's generally the case that a lot of women feel this way, that you have demands to live up to that you have to be there to such a degree that you tie yourself so closely to the children, see to their care and all this, so that you feel a great need to be yourself sometimes. And you can't do it in practice, because you're stopping yourself.

In this interpretation, the difference between them became a matter of fundamental disparities, he could not influence it; she had to do it herself.

These couples were successful in terms of achieving an equal division of labour. In the first couple, the division of labour was disadvantageous to her, whereas the division of labour was more equal in the second couple.

The differences in results depended, among other things, on the men's choice of different counter-strategies. In the one case, practical issues were turned into emotions, and the husband was quick to reconcile the issue. In terms of the practical issues themselves, none of them was willing to give in. In the second couple, the conflicts were transferred onto the children, and the couple's own relationship was not expressed in terms of conflicts. Regarding their differing standards of household and childcare, both parties made concessions to each other's demands, and both claimed that they had influence over the practical issues of their family governance. In her case, however, the need for self-governance and self-care had not been met. This had led to unresolved conflicts on her behalf. Both parties regarded these conflicts as internal, belonging to her. These inner conflicts were transferred onto the children, and caused conflicts with them. Her perspective of the self became characterised by self-sacrifice, and she did not find that acceptable. He was content with his strategies of self-governance, whereas she was discontented. In order for her to be content, it is probably necessary for her to assume a more reflexive approach to the duty norms that she lets herself be governed by.

Couples with strategies of subordination

We have identified some kind of subordination as a dominant strategy of conflict management in three couples. In these couples, the women perceived themselves as equal compared to their partners, despite the fact that they carried out significantly more work in the household. In two of the couples, the men had a dominating style and had retained their influence in decision-making, while the man in the third couple had chosen a subordinate stance by agreeing with his wife when she complained over his lack of engagement. He chose to be completely passive.

In the third couple, their mutual approach implied that the woman achieved what she wanted, and that she did not feel at all oppressed. This gave her a great deal of influence, but was also a heavy burden. It had developed into a long-drawn-out, ongoing process of conflict for her, since it seemed to be based on insufficient engagement for the jointly shared home on his behalf. It seemed to have led to a systematic delegation to her of all things related to the home and the family. She said:

> I have to start thinking about this and that a little earlier. And why should I be the one to think of the fact that we have to plan our vacation. I have to think ahead, e.g. that in this week, the child is going on an excursion, and the son needs to bring shoes – and he has none. I mean, how do I teach him that? It is not concrete, and it is very hard. But we could have, we could try, having long discussions that often end up with me becoming very irritated and I get furious, like. But then it's maybe better for a few

days. But as I said, the level gets raised eventually, but it happens very slowly.

The husband highlighted his own lack of engagement and claimed that she was more engaged, and thus also governed and made decisions 'since she is the more engaged and involved, then she's the one who . . . If something comes up, she is actually the one who knows better than me.' In his view, it seems as though her greater involvement meant that he should be less involved and engaged. Thus he chose not to compete or cooperate with her interests, but to subordinate any interests he might have in influencing his children, their consumption, holidays or economy.

Passivity or subordination became his counter-strategy, and her strategy of resistance expressed itself in countless discussions and sporadic emotional outbursts. The end result consisted in her giving up her demands and working for the communally shared. She gained a certain personal power from this, at the same time as she nourished a relational loyalty. His view was, however, that she did not have more influence over the household compared to him. According to our interpretation, he was unwilling to admit that he let himself be dominated, that he did not have a large say in many things in their daily existence, which can be difficult for a man to admit. It could also be difficult for him to admit that he enjoyed being dominated. There is an inherent ambivalence in this, but it could also entail comfort. Being dominated in the home can also be 'harmless', since the great passion was more oriented towards his work.

The other two couples differed, inasmuch as the men had significantly greater levels of influence and decision-making power over the division of labour in the household and the children. In both cases, the women argued that they did not feel subordinated, since the men made a bigger effort than they had expected – in one case, the man did more in order to feel independent, and in the other, she did more in order to be in control.

When the women in these couples described conflicts, they attributed themselves with a lack of ability to assert themselves using arguments. In one couple, the woman claimed:

> He is probably a little more dominating than me. More to the point and delivers quicker lines . . . he is more decided, has clear opinions straight away. When he has had his say, there is no room for discussion.

This type of argument reoccurred in the interview, when different situations were described. The husband was quick to assume a position, and cut off the discussion. The wife claimed that she was willing to listen to the husband's arguments, and would have liked him to listen to her as well. She described herself as 'not as clear in my thoughts, or as straightforward as him. He knows more, has a greater general knowledge.' In situations of conflict, they sometimes had it out and quarrelled loudly:

Yes, we raise our voices very much, and I often become sad and cry. Often I think he's wrong and he thinks I'm wrong, and nobody budges. We are equally stubborn.

The man said about himself:

I can be a little stubborn, so if I think something is good, I will push it through. Even if she is in doubt. I am a reflecting person, my opinions are clear; I speak them and speak them out straight.

He confirmed the picture of himself not only as the dominating person, but also as a person with self-confidence, who is not prepared to listen and discuss alternative viewpoints when he has contemplated and thought out where he stands. The reason why she would start crying was that she took things more personally, and she attributed her sensitivity to criticism because 'there has been a lot going on at work.'

The situation can also be interpreted as an expression of powerlessness, that his quick-paced and categorical approach left no room for her to express her opinion. The composite picture described by this couple was a conflict resolution type that began with competition – both maintained that their viewpoints were right. Subsequently, the conflict transferred her into a subordinating strategy, where she gave up and did not believe in the power of her own arguments, since she did not perceive them to be as well thought through as his, and because she did not have the ability to think clearly. Conversely, he claimed to be unable to discuss certain issues, such as housework, finances and so on. He maintained:

'I do not want discussions about these things, I get a stomachache from it, get irritated. I believe that there are at least two human beings, who fit together, and sometimes they get it right and then these conflicts are not necessary. If you have conflicts to start with, you might as well break up, you can't get to know each other.

To him, perceptions of housework are grounded in the personality, and impossible to change. While some opposing opinions are more or less grounded in thought-through arguments, others depended on personal attributes, which could not be discussed.

The woman in this couple let herself be governed by both obligations of care for the home and by his rights to define the situation. By subordinating her needs and interests, she came to reproduce an unselfish approach.

Also in this third couple, both parties described the man as a dominating person. However, the woman claimed to have developed personally – from having been very obliging to commanding respect. The change was precipitated by her acceptance of a managerial position at work, which forced her to make decisions and say how she wanted things. She transferred this way of relating to the family. Her story creates a picture of a woman in motion from subordination to a lesser acceptance of this subordination. She no longer accepted being dominated, and her strategy was to find her way to self-respect outside the communally shared sphere. There were several such elements in her story – she claimed that she hid her own 'luxury consumption', she questioned his way of directing her to be a mother according to a model that was not her own. She had therefore also chosen to speak her mind and assert her will to a greater extent, and had gained more self-respect that way. Her strategy to transgress the role patterns was characterised by ambivalence and reflection. She managed oppositions in the relationship not only by respecting his demands and being attentive to his needs, but also by being attentive to her own needs and demands. By addressing her own needs, she posed boundaries for how far his needs could trespass hers. After many years, she had thus been able to move from a self-sacrificing approach to a self-authentic approach.

Couples who avoid conflicts

In the couples who exemplify an avoiding strategy, both parties entertained the basic notion that the jointly shared budget was the most important aspect of the relationship. This related to everything – the finances, the household and the children. They presented themselves as a team, as a working entity that was upheld by work ethics, and this included the children, too. Everybody had to contribute to the jointly shared economy. For instance, this meant that one person should not be relaxing when another was working towards the common good. Both parties claimed to be quick to compromise. The husband pointed out that equality is fundamentally related to autonomy, being able to take care of yourself and be independent. This was equally important to the wife. Both parties stated that conflicts were extremely rare between them, but that they had a 'watch' on each other. They avoided open conflicts and chose to have a cohesive relationship. However, 'triangulations' could take shape within the family, where one parent or child was left out. This usually led to an outburst of emotion, which was swiftly subdued and referred to as 'loud discussions'. They were not perceived as conflicts – since this was threatening to both parties. The discussions were described as airing of opinions, not as opposing wills. Tensions were smoothed over, and evolved into avoiding strategies aimed at reinstating the harmony in the family. Maintaining the relationship became more important than discussing the issue at stake. In this case, relational ethics were given priority over problem-solving. None of them articulated their own needs.

Couples who cooperate

Among all interviews in the study there were only a few couples who described their togetherness according to a pattern that we perceive as cooperative. The couples we have chosen to illustrate this uphold independence and togetherness as supreme values. They have described their models of divisions of labour in accordance with what we refer to as the needs-oriented strategy. To the man, it was important to be competent in all areas, including caring for the home. He was keen on being involved and spending time with the child.

The woman emphasised that she wanted to secure her right to choose her own life, and forcefully defended the personal autonomy in their togetherness. It seems as though the couple had found a form that provided greater room for equality compared to the other couples in the study.

This couple claimed that conflicts regarding money, division of labour and views on child-rearing were rare. Both parties stated that they had firm rules regarding certain day-to-day routines, and much of this orbited around their child. The woman said: 'She [the child] governs our whole lives . . . but it's the most fun thing we have, it's the best we know, it's not negative.' Both parties tried as hard as they could to organise their work schedule so that somebody was always at home when their daughter came home after school. They had fixed rules regarding homework, and kept track of the demands the teacher made on the daughter's studies and other school-related matters. They also had a fixed mealtime routine. The husband said: 'When it comes to her [the child] we try to keep fixed bedtimes.' Both agreed that they did not have different views in terms of relating to the child or other interests. The woman claimed: 'When it comes to the child, we never disagree. We never disagree on financial matters, our daily life or if we are travelling somewhere.' Both stated that the woman was more of a driving force in terms of initiatives to make purchases or travels, whereas the man was more of an inhibiting force. Examples provided by both parties separately were identical, and their versions of decision-making processes corresponded. She had had a certain opinion that she pursued, and he pursued another. Both had retracted parts of their demands, and compromised in order to reach a decision that they both found acceptable. The woman said that she liked to have the last word, but in the examples given, it seemed as though no one always had the last word. She reacted negatively to the win–lose philosophy, which is implicitly inherent in the issue of having the last word:

> I say that in reality, we don't apply that style to get the last word like that. I think there is less and less fighting as the years go by. You find each other all the time. We know what our limits are and you don't overstep them like that. We don't provoke each other like that.

The man said that they did not have any conflicts, meaning that they do not shout forcefully at each other. However, they could disagree. In their descriptions on how they had arrived at solutions to tensions, factual arguments won either person over, and a solution was found.

Both parties had strong personalities, and in the interview they gave examples of behaviours that showed that they were prepared to drive their will through. Our interpretation of this couple relationship is that it exemplifies mutuality – being aware of your own needs and simultaneously be attentive to the needs of the other person. They exposed their boundaries and invited the other person to participate, but respected any rejections. Having had strong individual orientations also in the early stages of the relationship, they had developed towards a strong togetherness that built on respect for each other's needs and terms. The solutions they reached by discussion were, however, not based on deprioritising their own needs, but rather on sharpening the boundaries in regards to how far each party was prepared to adjust them.

Concluding comments

In this chapter, we have presented samples of how tensions were handled and how the couples have tried to pose boundaries for their self and others in the family. Scrutiny of the couples' different ways of managing these oppositions and posing boundaries indicate complex patterns. The examples also highlight the dynamics in the styles – strategies that are transformed over the course of the conflict. In several of the examples described, the actual conflict was not subject to resolution, but was transformed into something else, that could be managed.

In our analysis, we tested our classification of couples with different conflict management strategies against the models of division of labour that were identified in Chapter 6 – the *contract-oriented division of labour* that relies on agreements, the *needs-oriented division of labour* and the *characteristic gender-based division of labour* (approximately equal amounts in each group). We anticipated that among the couples where attempts at reaching agreements were a central theme for one or both parties, the strategies would be predominantly competing or cooperative. Couples with a needs-oriented division of labour had less emphasis on aspects of communication, since these models were described as operating on the needs recognised by each person, without necessitating detailed discussion. This model implies that opposing views are perhaps more difficult to acknowledge by the partners, for whom consequently avoiding or subordination would be more common strategies. In the third group of couples, both parties usually have determined opinions on division of labour, but the women in several cases attempted to persuade the husband to help out. In this case, we anticipated that the strategies applied would be characterised by subordination to a greater extent.

Among couples with a contract-oriented division of labour, applied by at least the woman, we found several strategies for managing tensions and posing boundaries. We found those with competing strategies, those who aimed at cooperation or compromise, and those who applied some form of subordination. Among the couples who were perceived to have a needs-oriented division of labour, we found two types of strategies in terms of managing differences in opinions when it came to the children or influence in the family – one characterised by cooperation and autonomy, and one characterised by male dominance and female subordination. Among couples with traditional divisions of labour, we also found communicative styles, but subordinating strategies were predominant. We are thus unable to draw any conclusions based on our sample regarding the communicative strategies used to manage tensions in reference to the overarching model of ideal and practice in terms of division of labour. We are also unable to see any difference between couples where men and women have equal socio-economic positions. Our material is qualitative, and can thus not be used for such an analysis with statistical reliability.

A vital reason why tensions are difficult to overcome lies in the powerful influence that operates on the basis of normative patterns that the women let themselves be governed by. The normative influence that ensnares the women functions as an effective blockade in all types of communicative strategies. We have also observed that men are alien to the same kind of normative governance and are unable to identify with it. They perceived the differences between the genders' perceptions of duties and 'musts' as stemming from the women's personalities and thus impossible to bring to battle. Even if the women succeeded in gaining substantial influence in the family, they still fall into patterns where they are hesitant, persuasive, perhaps nagging and emotional. These patterns are replicated when it comes to the children, purchases for the home and for themselves. The purpose of the patterns is to consolidate positions and decisions, and make sure everyone comes along. This type of tactic is identified as female ambivalence, and often lacks in authority both among men and the women themselves. Therefore, it does not hold its own in negotiations, or not even in cooperative strategies, since these require clear boundaries in terms of both parties' needs and interests. The men's communicative style may appear to be more factual and authoritative. Some avoid the factual issue and participate fully in the women's complaints, or refrain from listening. This does not lead to resolution of the conflict, however.

Chapter 9

The multifaceted gender equality

A complex picture

Judging from our results, both genders maintain equality as an ideal, or at least a normative guidance for togetherness. Men claim that equality is desirable, and the majority of them are prepared to contribute to and take part in the common care of the household. We have also been able to ascertain that it is mainly women who drive the achievement of equality forward. Even women who have a traditional view (often shared with their husbands) of the home as mainly a female responsibility, urge their men towards an increased participation, and the men must somehow meet the demands or wishes directed at them.

Our interviews with men and women about how they have come to solutions in regards to division of household labour, incomes and expenditure, ownership and savings and how they manage conflicts in their relationships relative to the children and other interests – have provided us with a complex picture – a multi-faceted image of equality, both as an ideal and in practice. We have found that in all couples, the women (mothers) shouldered the main responsibility for matters concerning the home, particularly in terms of household labour and childcare, irrespective of how much time they spend in paid work. These results correspond with most studies in this field. Within the frame of this main responsibility, there are many variations of approach to the division of labour in the family, however. The responsibility to administer the economy rests chiefly with the women, but the control of the economy lies often with both or only the men.

The rhetoric on equality consists of many varied perceptions of equality and what is ideal. Despite existing examples of conflicts and obvious injustices in how the couples divide labour and money, both men and women perceive themselves as equal. This is connected to the fact that the judgements are based on several criteria, and that different spheres in the relationship are weighed against each other. One can feel equal because both parties take responsibility for the jointly shared, regardless of whether the result of the division of labour is fair from a sameness perspective. One can feel equal because agreements are made and unnecessary conflicts are thus avoided, or because less pleasurable tasks can be swapped with more pleasurable tasks through such agreements. One can also feel equal because the belief is that things will even out in the long run.

However, we have not found that equality is associated with effectiveness or that perceptions of justice are not a living feature of perceptions of equality (Bäck-Wiklund and Bergsten 1997). Granted, the couples strive towards finding practical solutions, but pleasure and displeasure constitute a more significant factor in the division of domestic work than rationality or competence.

The complexity picture is strengthened by our inability to find any associations between division of labour and allocation of money. It is imaginable that couples who advocate agreements for division of labour would also have advocated more differentiated models for allocation of money. Differing between the separate and the jointly shared would for instance be conciliatory with the type of togetherness formed in relationships that feature open negotiations concerning your work and my work, my money and your money, my needs and interests and your needs and interests. However, we have found that the couples apply different principles and models of negotiation in relation to money and division of domestic work and care. For example, couples who divide labour strictly have also advocated strongly for and applied a joint economy, and vice versa.

It is clear that equality, as it is perceived on a day-to-day basis, is very remote from the ideal of sameness in sharing, which is the most common viewpoint represented in the public discourses on equality.

Initially, we stated that the change in the division of responsibility in the home is a slow process, but that changes still take place. We regard the fragmentary pattern that emerged from our results as an expression of a transformational process taking place within families, an increase in diversity of lifestyles, which also implies experimentation with new and tentative combinations. On a deeper level, this transformation can be seen as an identity crisis of couple relationships, against the background of previous generations' way of family life (Dubar 2000). It is obvious that male dominance in societal and family life, which for decades has been taken for granted both culturally and structurally, is in a state of dissolution. Subsequently, a crisis for both women and men ensues. The crisis viewpoint can be negatively interpreted. The negativity is related to an insecurity in relation to what the crisis may bring and to a lack of confidence in what the transformation may leave behind.[1] Insecurity and continuous testing of new approaches are inherent in crises. There is also a positive aspect to this, in that it may bear a promise of something new and better.

In this chapter, we will summarise and discuss the results in relation to our main themes, i.e. togetherness, autonomy and equality. Our purpose is to problematise the interaction between the concepts by making connections to the theoretical bases presented in Chapters 2, 3 and 4. In relation to these bases, we initially stated that we chose to study equality as a combination of the couples' own perceptions and the criteria used in the analysis: mutual balance in terms of division of resources and labour; space for self-governance and influence in conflict management, power and influence. One question we asked was: how do men and women in couple relationships practise and justify their division of labour, time, money and influence? This question was combined with the following question: how do couples create togetherness or family culture? We made the assumption that types of togetherness are associated with understanding of justice and equality. Equality and togetherness are also associated with individual boundaries and how couples manage conflicts or tensions in terms of interests and perceptions of relationship rules regarding division of labour, consumption and relationships with the children. The interaction between the individual, togetherness and equality are thus the central concepts applied in our analysis. How the couples understand and put these concepts into practice is not gender-neutral. In our analyses, we have referred to the significance of 'doing gender' for strategies of equality. From a wider perspective, this knowledge is of interest for the question of how and under what circumstances women and men reproduce, break or transgress gender norms.

This concluding discussion opens with a section about *equality and togetherness*. The overarching question addresses whether the shape of family togetherness is important for the shape of equality in divisions of labour and allocation of money. We will also discuss the relationship between patterns of division of labour and allocation of money based on its role in the togetherness.

In the following section, we will discuss the relationship between *autonomy and equality*. The purpose is to clarify the ways in which autonomy takes shape and what significance it has for equality in couple relationships.

Furthermore, we will discuss the relationship between methods of posing boundaries and managing tensions, and what these methods imply for the striving towards achieving changes in the gender relationships. We will revisit theoretical discussions and empirical evidence which aim to provide an understanding of how rigid structures are overcome. This discussion will bring us to a political level and the relationship between family and politics from a more overarching perspective. We will then conclude with a few highlights on family life, working life and equality as a political project.

In this summary, we will put greater emphasis on the female perspective. This is done since the tension between autonomy, equality and togetherness is more consciously managed by women in the home, because they are oriented towards change and are more reflexive in their approach.

Equality and togetherness

Equality is an ideal that actualises how utilities, work, money and influence are allocated using different forms of negotiation and concrete exchanges. Here, bargains are conducted and central resources such as pleasure and displeasure, competence, access to time etc. are balanced. Also included in this process is the interaction between different conflict management strategies, where different types of and approaches to power are central aspects. Through these strategies, different types of togetherness are formed and maintained. According to Fiske (1991, 1992), elementary forms of togetherness can be discerned (see Chapter 3). These are *communal sharing*, where the group is of superior importance; *calculating togetherness*, where the individual has a superior position; *equal balancing*, also oriented towards autonomy; and *authority ranking*, where togetherness is based on the person with the highest status in the group. As was described in Chapters 3 and 4, different forms of togetherness correspond to different principles of thought concerning morals and justice in relationships. Within the framework of these types of togetherness, we have discerned three main forms of division of labour. These consisted of a *contract-oriented* division of labour, where justice is viewed from the basis of sameness in distribution; a *needs-oriented* division of labour that applies a relational responsibility and a relationship-oriented justice thinking; and a *gender-based* division of labour where the justice thinking is based on status.

Togetherness and contract

The contract-based model of division of labour is associated with a calculating togetherness. This type of togetherness builds on agreements. The justice in this model relies on sameness in efforts by both parties, or on the existence of a reasonable relationship between give and take. The usual form for calculation, as expressed by the couples in terms of reasoning about divisions of labour, consists of pleasure and displeasure – bargaining for well-being or seeking to lessen one's discomfort with certain dislikes in the household work. The bargaining can also be about time – gaining time for one's interests, being able to do a good job or developing oneself.

Making deals about division of labour with or without calculations requires openness in speech about the issue. Style of negotiation, principles of justice and power are active elements in the creation of these contracts. As we have seen, it is not given that a contracts-oriented division of labour leads to equality in terms of sameness. This depends on how the parties evaluate the resources that are exchanged and how the process of conflict resolution is developed. The outcome can be like the couple in Hochschild's (1989) study, where the woman took the ground floor and the man took the basement. We have witnessed many examples where division of labour or money is neither equal nor proportional for both parties.

The calculating togetherness created by a contracts-oriented model for allocating resources is also what Giddens (1992) claims to be characteristic of the pure relationship. Agreements are met and adhered to as long as they have legitimacy. The legitimacy is the binding factor of this type of togetherness, along with trust that the agreements are implemented.

We could establish that several couples reached agreements, but a majority of women and their husbands stated that most men did not implement their agreements.

According to our interpretation, this is based on a division of power that gives the men the right to make the terms for their engagement and participation – men take the right to break agreements if they think they cannot or need not adhere to them, for various reasons. In the daily stream of events and activities, new priorities of commitments are created. The partners may believe that the responsibility has been temporarily suspended, but after a while, one is confronted with the fact that the temporary actions have become permanent habits and routines. We will return to this interpretation in the section about the individual and equality.

There are many subtle mechanisms that contribute to the breaking of agreements. For example, looking at how the couples divide money and material things, we see that many couples had made agreements that functioned in the way that both parties had imagined. However, this was not true of all couples, and the outcome was not entirely just in several cases, if by justice we mean equal amount to each party. The outcome of allocation of money between the jointly shared and the separate further illustrated that the more separate the allocation – i.e. the greater the space for separate economic space – the more explicit the agreements. The examples show that there also are economic 'grey areas' that create fluid boundaries between what was agreed and what came to be applied in practice. 'Grey areas' concern matters which are not thought of as joint, and which arise in the day-to-day household expenditure such as presents. The person (normally the woman) who is responsible for household consumption also tends to involve her personal finances in this grey area. We have seen several examples of this, and Nyman's (2002) studies have also confirmed this.

One interpretation is that the calculating type of togetherness does not have vitality, because it lacks something fundamental. This interpretation is based on an analysis of family togetherness that differentiates between the core family and its periphery. According to this interpretation, a non-calculating core, which is based on a gift economy, is an important prerequisite for functioning family cohesion. This is characterised by a sense of deep togetherness – a quality that discerns a home from a household. The significance of the reasoning of this analysis is that a couple relationship that builds on calculating togetherness will lack an inner core. In this type of relationship, a structure takes shape that may lead to disintegration, conflict, tensions and fragmentation. The couple would thus lack the dimension that we have referred to as relational ethics, that the individuals do not protect the relationship. This would mean that each person would give priority to his or her rights and autonomy, rather than weighing them against the need for togetherness (Holter and Aarseth 1994; Einarsdottir 2002).

We want to argue with this interpretation. Togetherness that builds on a contract or calculations may be fragile, since they in most cases are based on an unequal distribution of power, in gender terms. Yet, a calculating togetherness does not in principle entail that the parties do not care about the relationship. Protecting the relationship does not necessarily imply that the boundaries between the self and others or between own needs and the needs of others are diffuse. It could also imply recognition of the terms of the self *and* those of others, i.e. boundaries are drawn around the self, but the responsiveness remains. We have seen this type of approach in some couples. We have also come across this approach in the cooperation-oriented conflict management style. This style implies that interests are articulated, and that the communication is open – a prerequisite for the calculating togetherness.

Making agreements means that open negotiations are held, and the process itself can be important for creating a feeling of being together. In the negotiation, both parties have to articulate their needs and interests, and argue in favour of them. This means that in the negotiation arguments and interests are weighed against each other. Regardless of the result of the negotiation, the relational ethics applied through mutual respect and some type of impartiality is significant in terms of perceived justice (Kellerhals et al. 1997). We have found some examples where both parties have conveyed that their picture of the negotiation is perceived as just. However, we have also found several examples of negotiations with elements of dominance and lack of respect.

Togetherness and need

The second type of division of labour identified through the couples' descriptions of their everyday practice is needs based. In some couples, we were also able to identify a needs-based orientation in terms of allocation of money. This gained expression through the perception that a joint economy was superior to a separate economy. A needs-oriented model is associated with a needs-based justice for allocation and relational ethics. The reciprocity in this model rests on what we refer to as the gift economy of love. Giving does not anticipate receiving, since calculations suppress the gift economy of love. Yet, the gift economy is also associated with debt. It is the relationship between gift and debt that gives raise to a social bonding, i.e. togetherness.

What type of togetherness does the needs-oriented allocation derive from? The couples with this type of allocation spoke in favour of a principle that gave premium to the common good – not weighing and measuring for equal distribution, both in terms of allocation of money and labour. Relational ethics were prominent attributes in these couples. However, relational ethics can be expressed in several ways. One approach is to favour the needs and interests of others over one's own, which signifies absorption into the jointly shared (self-sacrifice). Yet if everybody applies this principle, a family culture is developed that Fiske (1991, 1992) refers to as communal sharing. Everybody should serve the common good, and as long as this remains in focus, the legitimacy for this type of togetherness is maintained. Yet, it could also imply that everybody is concerned with the well-being of each other, and that the caring is mutual. Such an approach represents equal balancing. The needs-based model creates a feeling of equality although the division is not equal from a sameness perspective. A needs-based model of allocation can also be a fragile basis for togetherness. If responsibility and work lean towards the disadvantage of one party for too long, it can be a humiliating experience for the party who has to carry the load. The basic logic of this model is that the jointly shared has the highest priority, and that the commitment is mutual – a relationship-based loyalty. The gift and debt economy of love is actively present. We have found examples of women who have refrained from arguing with their husbands regarding their efforts for the jointly shared activities, since their viewpoint is that the men should be aware of what they should do themselves. If the husbands did not realise this, they left it be – the jointly shared was not negotiable, it was a given.

Togetherness and gender traditionalism

Even if gender was in no way absent in couples who applied the contract- or needs-based models of division, it was not as explicit as in couples with a gender traditional division. Gender-based division of labour is founded on the principle of complementary in terms of obligations and rights. All parties should accept obligations and rights as legitimate, which in turn require that they are fulfilled and that some kind of balance exists – a balance of equal merit. The gift and debt economy of love is also relevant in this type of relationship, which Giddens (1992) associates with the practical formulation of the romantic love ideal in terms of female subordination and male power. The togetherness upheld in couples with a traditional division is based on what Fiske (1991, 1992) refers to as 'authority ranking', where status plays a definitive role. In this case, status is connected to social gender, where men and women have different rights and obligations, but where all things male have a higher value. We witnessed the symbolisation of this kind of relationship in e.g. the models of money allocation, in which the husband controlled the money and shared if his wife asked for it, and the instances when he found her consumption to be acceptable. Gaining help with the household or be given money for personal consumption was received as a gift of love, as was giving help or money. The absence of help was perceived as a lack of love.

Negotiations aimed at making the family function as a whole were also conducted in couples with a gender-based division. In our study, we have seen several examples of women seeking relief, both pleading for and demanding participation from their men, although they were of the opinion that women should have the main responsibility for the home and the children. We were able to conclude that the majority of the discontented women could be found in this category. Building togetherness on the principles of rights and obligations also requires norms regarding reciprocity.

In sum, we can conclude that the three models of division that we have iden-tified all have advantages and disadvantages when it comes to the possibility of uniting equality and togetherness. The needs-based and the gender-traditional models are based on the idea that division happens 'spontaneously' (needs-based) or 'naturally' (traditional). It may appear as though these models are less communicative and that the risk for misunderstanding is therefore greater than in the contract-based model, where levels of communication are higher. However, this model provides a fragile base for togetherness, since agreements are not always implemented, thus undermining trust and mutual respect.

Autonomy and equality

In the introductory chapters in this book, we referred to the emphasis on indi-vidualisation as a prominent trait by many researchers in discussion regarding modernity. Individualisation varies in its expression in many spheres in society. In family and social laws, there is a deregulation of the institutionalised depend-ency relationships between the genders in the family. The individual is gaining his or her own rights as well as an independent position in relation to the fam-ily and society. Individualisation has also been expressed in terms of a new view of the content of intimate relationships. In Gidden's (1992) interpretation, the view of the relationship is described in terms of exchange and reciprocity – the 'pure relationship'. For those who live in a pure relationship, togetherness means a heightened awareness of one's own needs, and a more active view of mutuality. The pure relationship is free from externally moderated rights and obligations. Instead, it is created by the commitments of the parties and their choice to create togetherness based on reciprocity. In this perspective, equality between the genders is central. Creating equality in everyday life is therefore largely about 'doing gender', i.e. as a woman, rising out of the entrenchment in fixed gender norms that govern them on a more or less conscious level. This is no mean feat, since gender norms suffuse all activities in society. Even if formal differences between the genders have been removed, or rather, the removal of formally divisive hindrances against women's and men's possibilities to claim their social rights in several respects, informal mechanisms that lead to different conditions or possibilities remain. Breaking gender boundaries is also about overriding these informal mechanisms.

In this book, we have provided many examples of women who are governed by norms that dictate that they should have the main responsibility for the fam-ily, the children and the household. Yet, we have also seen examples of women who distance themselves from what they perceive as duties that subordinate their own needs and interests in relation to the responsibility for the jointly shared. We have witnessed several strategies that counteract the ensuing lack of autonomy. We will now discuss these strategies, which are gaining a central position in the family; governing the men on women's conditions; changing oneself and one's conditions; creating one's own space. We will also discuss the importance of self-governance, and how this expresses itself from a male and a female perspective through a number of themes that have emerged in the presentation of the results.

Self-governance and power

Gaining a central position in the family

In Chapter 5, we saw that some of the women who perform more household labour than their men have chosen to do this, for example by working part time. Their choices are motivated by a wish to be in control over the situation at home. Through this choice, the women can maintain a central position in the family, and govern the togetherness in the family. We regard this strategy as a way of gaining power – in the sense of being able to direct others. By spending time working in the home, being responsible for planning the children's activities, planning meals and consumption, they can also assert their own needs and interests, even if it means that their own needs have to be subordinated to the needs that can be identified as common or that of others. The level of subordination of own needs in relation to common needs can be regarded as a free choice (i.e. that they are able to make alternative choices). This strategy can be regarded as an expression of self-governance. In most cases, this choice implies that the husband gains significantly more economic power, since his income is most likely to be higher than hers. For equality to apply in terms of sameness criteria, the prerequisite would be that the allocation of money and saving also automatically leads to female independence. In the example used to illustrate this type of situation, we could establish that the husband had a significantly higher income, and that he also had full control over the finances. The wife claimed to be totally disconnected from the economic issues – something which she had let happen herself. At the same time, she claimed that the most important issue was that women should not become economically inferior in the relationship. Despite this ideal, she had subordinated her own needs to the needs of the jointly shared, not only in terms of time and personal ambitions, but also in regard to her own financial scope of action. She was aware that she had come to embody a lifestyle that she previously had dissociated herself from. She was also aware that she had entered a female trap, but claimed that she was economically equal in relation to her husband, due to the economic division that they had created in terms of ownership and saving. She was thus also on her way towards adapting her equality ideals to the practical reality she had chosen to live her life in. This example illustrates the ambivalent situation between power, self-governance and subordination that many women find themselves in, and which is illustrated in this book. For those who work part time based on their free choice, it is important to emphasise that it is a conscious priority made on their own behalf, i.e. it is important to emphasise self-governance and influence. This prioritising, however, gives rise to new ambivalence in terms of loss of personal economic self-governance. As we have seen, diminished self-governance can be compensated with control over the jointly shared pool on several levels – economically, emotionally and socially.

Governing the men on women's conditions

In Chapter 5, we gave numerous examples of how women take the initiative to urge their men to become more involved, by nagging, persuasion, tears, anger, etc. The strategy was often conducted in such a way that the women defined the norms for the order, i.e. they strived towards creating equality based on the norms of duty that they themselves were governed by as women. The man was supposed to be governed by the same norms as the woman. In general, these norms were not accepted by the man, but were norms that the woman wanted to apply in his house, and that he had to adapt to. This was perceived by the man as a way for her to gain power – not only should he perform a task that he disliked, but also he should be made to think like her in terms of work and responsibility. This is similar to the situation that many women have had to adapt to in the labour market, where the men's way of life is the norm. Women are governed to act and think as if they were living on male terms, since managers and male colleagues expect that. Not surprisingly, we found that the men retaliated. Several examples were provided – active resistance, such as displaying inability or unwillingness, setting a lower norm for orderliness, claiming incompetence, referring to energy consuming workload or shirking from household duties by being at work. Yet, there were also examples of men who redefined the situation and proclaimed their need for independence. They claimed that their participation in the household labour granted them self-governance. This reflexive approach was also exemplified in that their efforts had to be made on their own terms, and that they wanted respect for having transgressed male gender boundaries.

Changing oneself and one's conditions

We have seen several examples of women who have reflected upon their conditions and made decisions, which have implied adjusting their own needs and interests. The above example (part-time work) illustrates one of the most common choices made by women in order to manage the ambivalence. As we have seen, this type of strategy is associated with redefining the situation, so that the choice has the appearance of a free choice, made not only on behalf of the children – that the children have a need to spend more time at home and have more calm surroundings – but also on behalf of themselves.

Some women chose to change their surrounding circumstances and began working full time in order to strengthen their personal economic power and the family economy. However, we found examples where full-time work does not guarantee increased control over the ambivalence of being governed by duty norms and developing self-governance. Nor did the full-time work automatically lead to an increased participation in the household labour by the man.

Some women accepted and received household help at home from a close relative. This strategy meant that the women are not fundamentally shedding the duty norms that they feel governed by, but that they are given relief and support for their perception of the importance of these norms by their surroundings, and in practice they do not question the gender order.

Reflecting upon the self and one's approach to orderliness means to actively manage the norms that one feels governed by, and to settle into a new reality. This strategy was also witnessed in both men and women. It implied a mutual acceptance of both norms for how the tasks should be carried out, levels of orderliness and conditions for the general performance of the task – times, frequency etc. This strategy is a long-term compromising solution, where both parties make concessions of their needs and interests. Compromises thus mean that no party is fully satisfied, but they also imply an active approach. They can lead to processes of reflection where the thoughts and emotions of the ego in relation to its needs and interests continue to be worked through.

Reflecting on different ways of managing conflicts also implies posing boundaries for the self and its interest and needs. Some women mentioned that they have altered their emotional approach to conflict management. To some, this has meant an improved ability to handle the issues and to pose boundaries for their needs and interests, thus leading to increased self-respect. Some have kept the lid on and avoided solving the conflict actively. This strategy may lead them into the next strategy for control – creation of their own space.

Creating one's own space

We have in different contexts heard women's stories about how they create room for their own interests in the jointly shared space. In the section about money, and in Chapter 8, we illustrated how women have created economic control over the household, how they have created space for their own time and in order to assert their approach to the children when parenting styles have diverged among the parties. Below, we will illustrate and discuss these strategies. In our encounters with the couples, we have come across women who have chosen a strategy to gain *control* over the household budget. These women saved money, mainly from their own incomes, but also from child allowances, and some from the money given to them by their parents. By splitting incomes into different accounts, they could conceal their own consumption or savings from the husband. The saving was combined not only with rationalised shopping styles and bargain hunting, but also with low levels of personal consumption. Strikingly, the main purpose of this was to create a buffer for the home and the children, but also for vacations and other shared activities. Since the women usually earned less, they had lesser amounts to operate with. Therefore, they were anxious to have the approval of their men for common purchases. By having money saved on their own account, they created a better negotiating position for themselves. Women had the power to tell the men to 'go to hell', as one man drastically put it.

We encountered several women who strongly emphasised their need for having time to themselves. In principle, we encountered no men who spoke about time in the same way as the women did. From the women's narratives, it was clear that what they wished for was time to take care of themselves and feel free from duties, being able to recharge and have space for reflection. In our culture, freedom is associated with autonomy and individualism. The implications of autonomy, in the male cultural tradition, are independence and freedom for action according to one's own goals, as well as the ability to choose without being hindered by the consideration for others as well as having alternative scopes of action. Autonomy is associated with a male understanding, which equals it with emotional and financial self-sufficiency. Autonomy means not needing anyone, but being able to manage on your own (Benhabib 1992). The implication of freedom offered by the women was not the same as the autonomy described above. The women spoke about being able to govern their lives in their own way. This meant being free from demands and duties – and not becoming completely exposed to other close relationships that simultaneously meant a lot to them. In this case, autonomy is associated with authenticity, not giving oneself up for the needs of others. Sacrificing yourself for others in order to gain acceptance means that parts of the self are denied. In the long run, this leads to low self-esteem. This is what the women speak about in terms of freedom.

In the section on women's approach to the children, we discussed the more regulating approaches that were regarded by men as correct, and the more argumentative style applied by the women. The couples provided several examples of how their different styles could lead to conflicts. In several cases, we could conclude that the women chose not to confront the men about these differences, but prevailed in their own style towards the children when the fathers were not present. In these cases, there was an obvious issue of ambivalence, since they 'publicly' accepted his interpretation of her style as being lax and unclear, whereas she remained true to her conviction of the right style for her and the children. The strategy can in itself be regarded as avoiding and reproductive of the male norm for how children should be treated. However, the discrepancy of their approaches was apparent, and several women chose to hold on to their own convictions, that is, to be authentic.

What do these different strategies mean in terms of self-governance and power in everyday practice? Are they sustainable in terms of the transformation of gender boundaries, or do they imply a reproduction of gender patterns? The answer to this question depends on if you apply the external or internal perspectives to judge equality, as discussed in Chapter 2. We will continue this discussion in the following section.

Transgressing gender boundaries

In our approach to the overarching question about the relationship between autonomy and togetherness on the one hand and equality on the other, we are now approaching the critical point of conclusion regarding the results that we have found. We have written about slow, yet possible changes towards equality of the genders in family life, and we have written about the relationship between autonomy and togetherness in the creation of more equal relationships between men and women in the family. The slow processes and the difficult transformation of the hierarchical relationship between the genders in the family have been attributed to the problems of being an individual who is working against the dominating cultural norms that guard the actions and priorities made in the day-to-day couple relationship practice.

In her book *Being Human: The Problem of Agency*, Margaret Archer (2000) presents a theory that concerns the transformational power of the individual.[2] It is difficult to summarise Archer's theory and her detailed conceptual clarifications in a few lines, but for our purpose, we will highlight a few central points in her theory.

First, she claims that life is always about predicaments, i.e. in life, the individual is confronted with tasks and problems that have to be solved. Second, she claims that emotions are an integral part in the theory of human agency, and form an all-encompassing and fundamental element thereof. Emotions are treated as sociological facts, and not as irrational and inner experiences that are hard to grasp. Emotions are defined as 'comments to our concerns' and are central factors of the predicaments that we handle in our everyday lives. This handling takes place through an inner dialogue of the individual. In this inner dialogue, emotions and rationality are thus united, i.e. the logical and factual is combined with emotional reasoning. A third central part of the theory is that the inner dialogue makes the self assume a position, and perhaps re-evaluates itself in relation to tasks and problems. This positioning is connected to the individual's self-perception and self-esteem. When assuming a position, one does so both sensibly and emotionally – thus entering a commitment. This means that the individual has re-evaluated his or her self, making a commitment built upon strong belief and loyalty. This choice is based on emotional and rational consideration.

Focusing on the instrumental and rational aspects in the negotiations with the self does not lead particularly far. To the singular individual, it is rather a matter of identifying the feelings experienced in relation to the object of negotiation, as a first step. The next step consists of considering what is particularly important, what one is prepared to put up with. The individual creates a preliminary rank order of the importance of the issues at stake. Following on this, the individual examines the costs of continuing as before or trying to change. The self conducts an inner conversation with itself about how it should relate to its position. The goal is to create 'solidarity' between you, and me where 'you' is the future self – the self that is aspired for, the self that the individual who is discontented in the present wants to become in the future. This means creating an authentic self. The third step revolves around making a decision that one is fully dedicated to. This implies that the individual must both prioritise and create ethics to adhere to.

Archer's (2000) train of thought is about how the individual changes his or her way of being and acting. Such a change is connected to the individual's identity. The focus is thus on the individual. One theme in this book concerns how individuals attempt to create change in an interpersonal gender order, particularly how women have tried to create changes in their men. According to Archer's reasoning, it is not possible for an individual to create a change of this kind in somebody else. The self changes only on its own accord. This means that the relationship can be changed by changing the self. When the self has changed, the other person in the relationship will have to relate to a different person. This predicament must be managed through an inner dialogue, in Archer's terminology. It is women in their day-to-day lives who experience this discrepancy between ideal and reality more profoundly. Women have the strongest motives to accomplish change, and it is women's actions that drive change forward. In other words, it is up to the women to change themselves in order to reduce the strength of normative power over the self, and change the ego towards a higher level of individualism, as was referred to above – towards increased authenticity. This requires posing of boundaries for their own actions, being more true to the self and one's interests and needs. Embedded in this is also the ability to discern the seemingly liberating strategies – which in fact reproduce old patterns – and locate the strategies that lead to actual transformation. By subordinating one's needs and interests in negotiations, or by avoiding communication, the risk ensues of creating a short-lived solution, which in the long term perpetuates the very patterns one wishes to break free from. Conflict resolution strategies that are aimed at cooperation or compromise, where one is forced to articulate one's interests and listen to the other person, provide promising prospects for this labour. An important consequence of this reasoning is also that negotiations about division of labour in the home must be held using both emotional and rational arguments. The solutions one has created will not be sustainable unless also the emotional aspects have been taken into consideration. This is perhaps why pleasure and displeasure are such important factors in the couples' negotiations.

The individual man and woman have to feel like the creator of his or her self. In our study, we have seen several examples of how women have developed strategies for self-governance, which we regard as expressions of reflection and authenticity. By choosing to be more authentic, men and women initiate a process where their partners also must confront the discrepancy between expectations and reality – this is the starting point for reflection, and in the long term also for change of their own approach.

We are of course aware that this is no simple process, and that it is loaded with powerful counter-reactions from the surroundings. According to the theory of 'doing gender', a person is held responsible for his or her choice of actions if they challenge normative expectations on gender. This is true for both men and women, but for women the process is heavier, since their position is inferior.

Nicky le Feuvre (1999) has studied women in professional careers, and how they have related to their female identities during these careers. Her findings show that breaks in the life course, in addition to what the career itself has brought with it, often lead to reflection and re-evaluation of one's existence as a woman. These women have been able to transform their gender identity. Other women in their careers have given up their identity and assumed male gender norms. She also found examples of women who have adapted and simply reproduced their way of being a woman (le Feuvre 1999).

It is within the framework of these ways of reasoning that we can manage the answers to the questions of what strategies lead to the reproduction of gender orders on the interpersonal level. The effects of these strategies on the subjective level are most relevant in terms of how the conflict resolution will progress. The individuals in the couple have a shared history, a future to handle – the present may seem static to the observer on the outside. It does not follow that one strategy freezes the gender positions in the couples for the rest of their lives. There are more examples of how the couples have changed – but also examples that show that they have not.

Epilogue

We cannot conclude this book with the singular argument that women and men must individually change their attitudes towards the normative gender guidelines that they more or less consciously are engrossed by in their everyday lives. Even if each individual has to take a stand for changes made in his or her own life, there is also a joint responsibility on a societal level for contributing to changed relationships between the genders.

One of the questions raised in this study is how we can understand the slow processes of change in the gender division of responsibility for the home, the children and family relations. In the public discourse, discussions on gender equality focus on gender inequality, rather than on what gender equality means in practice. One purpose of this study was thus to relate men's and women's understanding of gender equality to the understanding of equality that is discussed on a political level. The results show that there are wide discrepancies between marriage partners in how they understand equality, and that these variations are associated with how they manage the relationship between autonomy and togetherness. In the political discourse on gender equality, a central dimension in the policy has been to strengthen women's independence of family and husband in terms of sustenance. This has been achieved partly by emphasising the equality between the spouses in marital law, and partly by creating conditions on which women can sustain themselves. Through individual taxation and individual social rights in social insurance, the individual's responsibility for his or her own sustenance has been emphasised. Of particular importance in this context are the parental insurance and the expansion of public childcare.

Several political actions have thus been of great significance for strengthening the rights of the individual in the family and society. These actions have been significant markers for gender equality, both culturally and normatively. The politics has been steadfast in creating justice and equal conditions for negotiations in families regarding the division of labour between the genders. Gender equality in the policy context has largely been understood in terms of sameness and proportionality. However, as the study shows, autonomy and independence represent one side of equality, while togetherness and mutuality represent another side. This and many other studies of family and division of labour between the genders show that women carry the main responsibility for the home, the children and the family – and women are the ones who create togetherness. To an increasing extent, women's commitment and responsibility for these activities is paid for by their health.

Since the mid-1970s, the political debate in Sweden has mainly given its attention to the unequal terms of working life. This is associated with the fact that many reports have revealed that the development towards gender equality in working life is not progressing according to expected time-frames. A government report on the power of women published in 1997 (Swedish Government Official Reports Series 1998: 6) gave numerous indications that women's conditions in working life are worse than men's on several counts. Various reports on changes in the welfare system during the 1990s show that the levels of stress in female-dominated professions have increased markedly since the 1980s. Stress has also increased in male-dominated professions during the same period, but not to the same extent as in the female-dominated professions. The greatest increase has taken place in care professions, education and retail, i.e. in professions that are characterised by relationships and care. In some female-dominated professions, the portion of stressful work was as high as 80 per cent. In these sectors, both the working environment and the relative wage levels have worsened drastically. The increase in women's educational level during the same period has not been followed by a corresponding increase in their wages (Swedish Government Official Reports Series 2000: 3, Fritzell et al. 2001; Swedish Government Official Reports Series 2001: 79).

The survey that formed the basis for this study showed a clear connection between stress in working life and stress in the home. Furthermore, the investigation showed that there was an association between perceived health and conflicts regarding domestic work. Conflicts give rise to more stress and worse health. Women's health is generally worse than men's health. Prevalence of women's sick leave has increased markedly since the beginning of the 1990s. The increase in illness is largely due to increased stress in working life. However, since there is an association between perceived stress at work and in the home, there is reason to consider the unequal gender relations in families as a health problem for women (Björnberg 1998).

The structures in working life that create and maintain unequal terms for women are connected with the division of labour in the family. The family structure interacts with several other societal structures – structures that create gender segregation and discrimination in regards to wages and working conditions. In different ways, these structures perpetuate the conditions for women and men in working life and in politics. The labour market and the gender relations that are active within it have been adapted to the reforms aimed at supporting women's wage labour. Certain working life niches have been created for women, where adjustments have been made to pregnancy and having children, and to the fact that women care for children and take long periods of parental leave. In these female-dominated workplaces, there are routines for managing women's wish to work part time. Wages and career opportunities have been adjusted so that the wages are lower and the jobs do not provide any major career opportunities. This is often attributed to the fact that women have the main responsibility for the home and family (Björnberg 2002). In male-dominated workplaces, it is taken for granted that the women take parental leave, and men take only a fraction of the leave, if any (Hwang 2000). As in society at large, the gender order in the family operates through the division of labour, chiefly connected to the children, which gives women the main responsibility for the unpaid labour, gives them lower wages and worse working conditions.

The work that women do in families renders them a lower market value, since care and social reproduction is of low economic and social value in society (but not necessarily personal). This low evaluation has deep political-philosophical roots, and can be illuminated with reference to the relationship between justice ethics and care ethics, as viewed from a societal perspective. In her analysis of the meaning of these concepts, Selma Sevenhuijsen (1998) claims that society incorporates a structural conflict between principles of civil rights to freedom and autonomy (and thus also justice ethics) on the one hand, and care ethics connected to dependency and limitations of the individual's options on the other.

She claims that in western society, there is a superior tendency to think in terms of dualism. Concepts such as male and female, fatherhood and mother-hood, culture and nature, rationality and emotionality, body and soul, public and private, universal and particular are examples of this. In each representa-tion of such dualistic concepts, there is a hierarchy which is maintained by the definition of one as more valuable or superior to the other, which is less valu-able or inferior. If applied to justice ethics and care ethics, the justice ethics are regarded as more valuable than ethics that are associated with relationships, care and dependency.

The discourses on justice ethics and care ethics represent cultural norms that give structure to how we think, act and make judgements. Carol Gilligan (1982) gives examples of this in her studies on ethical principles. She argues that those who make arguments with reference to justice and individuality were perceived as representing a higher level of maturity than those who make arguments with reference to care for relationships and that which promotes togetherness. There are several other examples of how care represents a low value; e.g. the wage levels in care professions, or the perception that domestic work is boring or unpleasant – a necessary evil that couples negotiate about, with pleasure and displeasure as trading currencies.

The relationship between justice ethics and care/relational ethics has been the topic of many discussions in feminist research (see for example Okin 1989; Benhabib, 1992). According to Sevenhuijsen (1998), there is a normative fault in the feminist discourse on care ethics. This is due to the fact that care in this con-text has been associated more with morals and less with actual activity. Care has come to be understood in the context of motherhood and femininity, which is associated with good, altruism and dependence. Sevenhuijsen criticises the feminists (standpoint feminists) who want to emphasise that care is a particular female activity, and that care ethics represents a female ethics with a higher value than justice ethics. These feminists have merely chosen to reverse the hierarchical order without questioning its basis. Care ethics does not represent a specifically female moral, according to Sevenhuijsen. Care is primarily a social practice, and not a moral activity. Care is directed not only at others, but also towards the self – i.e. something which affirms the individual as an autonomous person. Care exists not only in the family, but also in several types of relationships – at work, in friendship, etc. As a practice, care does not have only positive values. Relationships, dependencies and care should be acknowledged as ordinary, human values, and not as something that the autonomous, self-sufficient individual is free from.

Politics plays an important role in reminding the public of everybody's need to be part of relationships and dependencies. The solidarity which is created within the framework of social dependencies has a central value, and is neither opposed nor subordinated to the individual's rights and justice. In terms of social practice as activity, there is, however, also reason to scrutinise relational work as such, as well as its qualities and spread. In this study, we have been able to establish that it is mainly women who perceive the norms for domestic work and care for the home and the children as the most reasonable. An underlying judgement is that men should take on the same norms for the neat and well-maintained house, and if they do not, the women 'have to' show them the significance of these norms or do the cleaning and caring themselves. As such, care is generally a female occurrence, and not something that men want to identify with. Men's perceptions of norms that concern domestic work are rarely a matter of public discussion, and when discussions take place, they focus on flaws, faults, passivity and dissociation. Men's norms for the significance of everyday care of children is also rarely articulated in public, and when they are, they are often coupled with images of slightly helpless men in suits, holding a protesting baby in one arm and a mobile phone in the other. These various representations in the discourse both illustrate and contribute to the emphasis of different normative guidelines for femininity and masculinity without questioning them.

If we take a look at how both men and women prioritise their use of time, we may still be able to trace a change. Historical and internationally comparative studies have shown that women in general have reduced the time they spend in domestic work (excluding childcare), and that men use more time in such activities. Women and men have thus narrowed the gap between them (Gershuny 2000). These results can be interpreted so that women have come closer to male norms to a greater extent than vice versa, since women have reduced their time-use to a greater extent than the men have increased theirs. Gershuny has also found that in general, leisure time has increased. Despite the fact that the total time in wage labour tends to decrease, increasingly more individuals experience that they need to accomplish more in the twenty-four hours of the day. Time is filled with other types of activities, particularly for consumption of goods and services, according to Gershuny (2000). Certain services relieve or replace the individual's own time, while other services require input of own time, such as workouts, sports, learning and personal development. In the new economy, household consumption of services and goods is necessary for economic growth. Gösta Esping-Andersson (1999) draws similar conclusions in his book about the post-industrial economy. In order to live up to this development, time politics must also be developed, according to these researchers. The significance of time politics (e.g. shorter work hours, extended leaves to attend to issues related to the home) for the gender-equality perspective is an open question, however. Depending on how it would be formulated, it can promote gender-equality by dissolving the hierarchical dualism of work and private life. It may have the consequence that the home and private relationships no longer will be considered female activities of a lower value. Making parental insurance an individual right, where women and men are given an equal number of days which cannot (unlike the current system) be transferred to the other parent (usually the woman) is a possible measure that can be implemented to such an effect.

Notes

1 Introduction

1 The results from this study have been outlined in articles and book chapters (Björnberg 1996, 1997, 1998). A selection of results will also be presented along with the presentation of the qualitative study in this book.
2 The sample was random and included parents with children of pre-school age (approximate age 5 years) (Björnberg 1997); 60 per cent of these parents also had younger children below the age of 5 years. The sample was not nationwide, but restricted to rural and urban areas of west Sweden.
3 Most couples in the study were married, but some were cohabiting. We use the term 'partners' to cover both.
4 Five of twenty-two mothers were in paid work, between 70 and 90 per cent working full time; five of them worked half time. Ten of the women worked in the care sector, eight in other industries and four worked in the manufacturing industry. Fifteen of the men had service professions, mainly in the private sector, and seven were qualified workers. The husbands had higher levels of education than their wives in two cases, and the wives had higher levels of education than their husbands in four cases. In five of the couples, the partners had the same income, in four cases, the women had a higher income and in thirteen cases, the men had the higher income. A few couples were very homogenous in terms of profession, but the incomes were significantly different. Fourteen of the interviewed couples owned the property they lived in, and six were living in rented accommodation.

2 Gender equality in families

1 Our understanding of the concept 'adult worker family model' is basically that provision of material support is publicly expected (through tax rules and regulations of social benefits) by adult family members and that each partner is responsible for maintenance of themselves and members of the family with two generations, regardless of marriage or sex.
2 The Swedish welfare state has been portrayed as 'a social democratic model' primarily by Gösta Esping-Andersen (1990). Korpi (2000) prefers the term 'encompassing/dual-earner model', since there is no homogeneous social democratic model.
3 Additional child allowance is paid to those families with three or more children. For the third child an extra amount of 28 € a month is paid, for the fourth 83 € and then 104 € extra a month for the fifth and any following children (Swedish Government Official Reports Series 2001: 24).
4 The literature on sex and gender is currently very comprehensive. For a deeper orientation, we refer to Connell (1987), Magnusson (1998) and Hirdman (2001).

4 Negotiations, conditions and strategies

1 Kari Waerness (1987) distinguishes between care work and service work. Caring for a person who is dependent on support to manage everyday life is care work, whereas service work is carried out for individuals who are capable of managing their own needs.

2 Thylefors (1996: 102) differs between strategy, technique and tactics in conflict management. Strategy is used synonymously with style, and describes overarching approaches, e.g. compromise. Tactics represent how power and influence are used in the situation. Technique refers to singular efforts made in the negotiation, e.g. speech or action.

5 Division of labour in the household

1 It is possible that women report more conflicts than men. The difference between men and women who live together can in this case be attributed to the fact that more women than men were interviewed (309 versus 215).

2 We are not concerned here whether this couple should be regarded as 'equal' according to a predetermined definition. It is an interesting question, but not relevant to this study.

3 Einarsdottir (2002) maintains that the dual concepts of traditional–modern presuppose a dualistic view of history, in which the concept of traditional is associated with something inadequate, belonging to an earlier form of society. She therefore prefers to speak of a gender-complementary division of labour. Our position is that her criticism is justified, but we will continue to use the term 'traditional' varyingly and synonymously with the term gender-complementary.

4 One of the women wanted full-time work, but wasn't able to do so after a period of unemployment. The other woman could have worked part time, but not within the position that she preferred.

5 In the original survey, 25 per cent chose to take care of the children themselves. However, some of them had parental leave, and the survey does not reveal how many parents choose not to use nurseries.

6 How is equality in division of labour created?

1 Quoted in Lennéer-Axelson and Thylefors (1996: 264). Translator's adaptation into English.

7 Sharing and allocating money

1 In the investigation, this situation was referred to as 'economic deprivation'. The measure (PDI – Proportional Deprivation Index) was constructed so that the respondent allocated which items of consumption on a list of thirty-eight items were deemed by them as socially necessary, but not affordable to them. For a more detailed description of the PDI, see Halleröd (1995, 2001).

2 The couples that were classified as purely joint were couples in which both partners agreed that they were equally responsible for managing the economy of the household.

3 Parents, paid work and family policy, own data.

4 'Separate' and 'divided' are used as synonymous terms.

8 Posing boundaries and managing conflicts

1 It is highly subjective what different persons mean by conflict. Some give the term a wide meaning that includes differences in opinion, and disputes – implicit or explicit

– while others use the term only to describe outright quarrels. For an in-depth discussion about conflicts, see Lennéer-Axelsson and Thylefors (1996).
2   χ^2 strength of association p = 0.05.

9   The multifaceted gender equality
1   Fears are expressed that care and risk management, which are among the most vital functions of the family, are becoming increasingly hollow through the changes brought by the transformation of gender relations (see for example Castells 1997; Esping-Andersen 1999).
2   The book is the final one in a trilogy that delineates the relationship between structure, culture, nature and human action. For our purpose we have included an extract of selected parts of the comprehensive theory.

References

Agell, Anders (1998) *Äktenskap, samboende och partnerskap* (*Marriage, Cohabitation and Partnership*). Uppsala: Justus Förlag.

Ahrne, Göran and Roman, Christine (1997) *Hemmet, barnen och makten: Förhandlingar om arbete och pengar i familjen* (*Home, Children and Power: Negotiations on Work and Money in the Family*). SOU 1997: 139 (Swedish Government Official Reports Series. Stockholm: Statens offentliga utredningar (SOU).

Andersson, Gunnar (1993) *Leva för jobbet och jobba för livet: Om chefsfamiljers vardag och samlevnadsformer* (*Living for Work and Working for Life: About the Everyday Lives of Managers and their Families*). Stockholm: Brutus Östlings Förlag.

Anxo, Dominique (2003) 'Division sexuelles des tâches: les experiences françaises et suédoises' ('Gender division of domestic work: French and Swedish experiences'), in *Futuribles analyse et prospective*, 285 Avril: 33–41.

Archer, Margaret (2000) *Being Human: The Problem of Agency*. Cambridge: Cambridge University Press.

Attanucci, Jane (1988) 'In whose terms: a new perspective on self, role, and relationship', in *Mapping the Moral Domain*, (eds) Carol Gilligan, Janie Ward, and Jill McLean Taylor. Cambridge, MA: Harvard University Press.

Bäck-Wiklund, Margareta and Bergsten, Birgitta (1997) *Det moderna föräldraskapet: En studie av familj och kön i förändring* (*Modern parenthood: A Study of Changing Family and Gender.*) Stockholm: Natur och Kultur.

Beck, Ulrich and Beck-Gernsheim, Elisabeth (1995) *The Normal Chaos of Love*. Cambridge: Polity.

Becker, Gary (1993) *A Treatise on the Family*, enlarged edn. Cambridge, MA: Harvard University Press.

Benhabib, Seyla (1992) *Situating the Self: Gender, Community and Postmodernism in Contemporary Ethics*. Cambridge: Polity.

Berger, Peter and Kellner, Hansfried (1970 [1964]) 'Marriage and the construction of reality', in *Recent Sociology No. 2*, (ed.) Hans Peter Dreizel. London: Macmillan.

Bjerrum Nielsen, Harriet and Rudberg, Monica (1994) 'The cacophony of gender identity – an interlude', in *Psychological Gender and Modernity*, (eds) Harriet Bjerrum Nielsen and Monica Rudberg. Olso: Scandinavian University Press.

Björnberg, Ulla (1996) '*Living on the edge: lone mothers in the new Europe*' in TRANSFER. Quarterly of the European Trade Union Institute Vol 2 No 2 1996.

Björnberg, Ulla (1997) 'Swedish dual earner families: gender, class and policy', in *Families with Small Children in Eastern and Western Europe,* (eds.) Ulla Björnberg and J. Sass. Aldershot, UK: Ashgate.

Björnberg, Ulla (1998) 'Psychological well-being among women with preschool children' in *Women, Stress and Heart Disease*, (eds) Margaret Chesney, Kristina Orth-Gomér and Nanette Wenger. New York: Erlbaum.

Björnberg, Ulla (2002) 'Ideology and choice between work and care: Swedish family policy for working parents', *Critical Social Policy* 22(1): 33–52.

Bloch, François, Buisson, Monique and Mermet, Jean-Claude (1992) 'From dis-jointed to joint parenthood', in *One Parent Families*, (ed.) Ulla Björnberg. Amsterdam: SISWO.

Blumberg, Rae Lesser (1991) 'Introduction: the "Triple Overlap" of gender stratification, economy and the family', in *Gender, Family and Economy*, (ed.) Rae Lesser Blumberg. London: Sage.

Bolin, Kristian (1997) 'Familj, makt och ekonomiska resurser – den nya famil-jeekonomin', ('Family, power and economic resources – the new economy of families'), in *Familj, makt och jämställdhet (Family, Power and Equality)*, (eds) Göran Ahrne and Inga Persson. SOU 1997:138. (Swedish Government Official Reports Series). Stockholm: Statens offentliga utredningar.

Borchgrevink, Tordis (1995) 'The fearful empty space', in *Labour of Love: Beyond the Self-evidence of Everyday Life*, (eds) Tordis Borchgrevink and Œystein Gullvåg Holter. Aldershot: Avebury.

Bourdieu, P. (1999) *Den manliga dominansen (Male Dominance.)* Göteborg: Daidalos.

Burgess, Ernest W. and Locke, Harvey J. (1945) *The Family: From Institution to Companionship*. New York: American Book Company.

Castells, Manuel (1997) *The Power of Identity*. Cambridge, MA: Blackwell.

Chafetz, Janet Saltzman (1991) 'The gender division of labor and the reproduction of female disadvantage: toward an integrated theory', in *Gender, Family and Economy*, (ed.) Rae Lesser Blumberg. London: Sage.

Cheal, David (1988) *The Gift Economy*. London: Routledge.

Cheal, David (1991) *Family and the State of Theory*. New York: Harvester/Wheatsheaf.

Chronholm, Anders (2002) 'Which fathers use their rights? Swedish fathers who take parental leave?' *Community, Work and Family* 5(4): 365–370.

Clark, M. S. and Chrisman, K. (1995) 'Resource allocation in intimate relationships: trying to make sense of a confusing literature', in *Entitlement and the Affectional Bond: Justice in Close Relationships*, (eds) Melvin J. Lerner and Gerold Mikula. New York: Plenum Press.

Connell, R. W. (1987) *Gender and Power: Society, the Person and Sexual Politics*. Cambridge: Polity.

Crompton, Rosemary (ed.) (1999) *Restructuring Gender Relations and Employment: The Decline of the Male Breadwinner*. Oxford: Oxford University Press.

Daly, Mary (2000) *The Gender Division of Welfare: The Impact of the British and German Welfare States*. Cambridge: Cambridge University Press.

Dubar, Claude (2000) *La Crise des identités: l'interprétation d'une mutation (The Crisis of Identities: Interpreting a Transformation)*. Paris: Presses Universitaires de France.

Einarsdottir, Torgerdur (2002) 'Who rules in the core of the family?', in *Autonomy and Dependence in the Family: Turkey and Sweden in Critical Perspective*, (eds) Rita Liljeström and Elisabeth Özdalga. Transactions no. 11. Istanbul: The Swedish Research Institute in Istanbul.

Ekstam, K. (2000) *Handbok i Konflikthantering* (*Handbook of Conflict Management*). Malmö: Liber.

Elwin-Nowak, Ylva (1999) *Accompanied by guilt: Modern Motherhood the Swedish Way*. Stockholm: Department of Psychology, Stockholm University.

Esping-Andersen, Gösta (1999) *Social Foundations of Post-industrial Economies*. Oxford: Oxford University Press.

Fenstermacher, Sarah, West, Candace, and Zimmerman, Don H. (1991) 'Gender inequality: new conceptual terrain', in *Gender, Family and Economy*, (ed.) Rae Lesser Blumberg. London: Sage.

Finch, Janet (1989) *Family Obligations and Social Change*. London: Polity.

Finch, Janet and Mason, Jennifer (1993) *Negotiating Family Responsibilities*. London: Routledge.

Fiske, Allan Page (1991) *Structures of Social Life: The Four Elementary Forms of Human Relations*. New York: Free Press.

Fiske, Allan Page (1992) 'The four elementary forms of sociality: framework for a unified theory of social relations', *Psychological Review* 99: 689–723.

Fritzell, Johan, Gähler, Michael, and Lundberg, Olle (2001) *Välfärd och arbete i arbetslöshetens årtionde*. Kommittén Välfärdsbokslut. SOU 2001: 53 (Swedish Government Official Reports Series). Stockholm: Fritzes.

Fürst, Gunilla (2000) *Sweden: The Equal Way*. Stockholm: Svenska institutet (Swedish Institute).

Gaunt, Louise (1987) *Familjekretsen: bosättning, umgänge och omsorg.* (*The Family Circle: Settling, Interaction and Care*). Gävle: Statens institut för byggnadsforskning (National Institute for Building Research).

Gershuny, Jonathan (2000) *Changing Times: Work and Leisure in Postindustrial Society*. Oxford: Oxford University Press.

Giddens, Antony (1992) *The Transformation of Intimacy: Sexuality, Love and Eroticism in Modern Societies*. Cambridge: Polity.

Gilligan, Carol (1982) *In a Different Voice: Psychological Theory and Women's Development*. Cambridge, MA: Harvard University Press.

Gilligan, Carol (1988) 'Remapping the moral domain: new images of self in relationship', in *Mapping the Moral Domain*, (eds) Carol Gilligan, Janie Ward, and Jill McLean Taylor. Cambridge, MA: Harvard University Press.

Gilligan, Carol and Attanucci, Jane (1988) 'Two moral orientations', in *Mapping the Moral Domain* (eds) Carol Gilligan, Janie Ward and Jill McLean Taylor. Cambridge, MA: Harvard University Press.

Godbout, J. (1992) *L'Esprit du don* (*The Spirit of the Gift*). Paris: La Découverte.

Goodnow, Jacquelin J. and Bowes, Jennifer M. (1994) *Men, Women and Household Work*. Melbourne: Oxford University Press.

Gouldner, Alvin (1973) 'The norm of reciprocity', in *For Sociology: Renewal and Critique in Sociology Today*. London: Allen Lane.

Haavind, Hanne (1982) 'Makt og kjærlighet i ekteskap' ('Power and love in marriage'), in *Kvinneforskning: Bidrag til en samfunnsteori* (*Women Studies: Contribution to Social Theory*), (eds) R. Haukaa, M. Hoel and H. Haavind. Oslo: Universitetsförlaget.

Haavind, Hanne (1987) *Liten og stor: Mødres omsorg og barns utviklingsmuligheter* (*Small and Big: Mothers' Care and Children's Development Opportunities*). Oslo: Universitetsforlaget AS.

Halleröd, Björn (1995) 'The truly poor: indirect and direct measurement of consensual poverty in Sweden', *Journal of European Social Policy* 5(2): 111–129.

Halleröd, Björn (2001) 'Employment positions, class and economic hardship: a longitudinal study of labour market marginalization and consumption', in *Employment, Unemployment, Marginalisation*, (ed.) Bengt Furåker. Göteborg Studies in Sociology, no. 1. Göteborg: Department of Sociology, Göteborgs Universitet.

Hirdman, Yvonne (2001) *Genus – om det stabilas föränderliga former. (Gender – On Stability and its Changing Forms)*. Malmö: Liber.

Hochschild, Arlie Russell (1989) *The Second Shift: Working Parents and the Revolution at Home*. London: Piatkus.

Holmberg, Carin (1993) *Det kallas kärlek: En socialpsykologisk studie om kvinnors underordning och mäns överordning bland unga jämställda par (They Call it Love: A Social Psychological Study on Women's Subordination and Men's Power in Young Equal Couples)*. Göteborg: Anamma.

Holter, Øyvind Gullvåg and Aarseth, Helene (1994) *Mäns livssammanhang (Living Circumstances of Men)*. Stockholm: Bonnier utbildning.

Hörnqvist, Martin (1997) 'Familjeliv och arbetsmarknad för män och kvinnor' ('Family life and labour market for men and women'), in *Familj, makt och jämställdhet (Family, Power and Equality)*, (eds) Göran Ahrne and Inga Persson. SOU 1997: 138 (Swedish Government Official Reports Series). Stockholm: Statens offentliga utredningar.

Hwang, Philip (2000) 'Pappors engagemang i Hem och Barn' ('Dads' engagement in the home and the children'), in *Faderskap i Tid och Rum (Fatherhood in Time and Space)*, (ed.) Philip Hwang. Stockholm: Natur och Kultur.

Jónasdóttir, Anna (1991) *Love, Power and Political Interests: Towards a Theory of Patriarch in Contemporary Western Societies*. Örebro: Örebro Studies.

Júlíusdóttir, Sigrún (1993) *Den kapabla familjen i det isländska samhället: En studie om lojalitet, äktenskapsdynamik och psykosocial anpassning (The Capable Family in Icelandic Society: A Study on Loyalty, Marriage Dynamics and Psychosocial Adjustment)*. Göteborg and Reykjavik: Department of Social Work, Göteborg University.

Kaufmann, Jean-Claude (1992) *La Trame conjugale: analyse du couple par son linge (The Marriage Drama: Analysis of Couples through their Textiles)*. Paris: Nathan.

Kellerhals, Jean, Coenen-Huther, Jean, and Modak, Marianne (1988) *Figures de l'équité: la construction des normes de justice dans les groupes*. Paris: Presses Universitaires de France.

Kellerhals, Jean, Modak, Marianne, and Perrenoud, David (1997) *Le Sentiment de justice dans les relations sociales. (Sense of Justice in Social Relationships)*. Paris: Presses Universitaires de France.

Klein, David M. and White, James M. (1996) *Family Theories*. London: Sage.

Knudson-Martin, C. and Mahoney, A. R. (1998) 'Language and processes in the construction of equality in new marriages', *Family Relations* 47: 81–91.

Kollind, Anna-Karin (2002) *Äktenskap, konflikter och rådgivning: Från medling till samtalsterapi (Marriage, Conflicts and Counselling: From Mediation to Therapy)*. Stockholm: Carlsson Bokförlag.

Komter, Aafke E. (ed.) (1996) 'Introduction', in *The Gift: An Interdisciplinary Perspective*, (ed.) Aafte E. Komter. Amsterdam: Amsterdam University Press.

Korpi, Walter (2000) 'Faces of inequality: gender, class and patterns of inequalities in different types of welfare states', *Social Politics* 7(2): 127–192.

Kugelberg, Clarissa (1999) *Perceiving Motherhood and Fatherhood: Swedish Working Parents with Young Children*. Uppsala Studies in Cultural Anthropology no. 26. Uppsala: Acta Universitatis Upsaliensis.

Le Feuvre, Nicky (1999) 'Gender, occupational feminization, and reflexivity: a cross-national perspective', in *Restructuring Gender Relations and Employment: The Decline of the Male Breadwinner*, (ed.) Rosemary Crompton. Oxford: Oxford University Press.

Lennéer-Axelsson, Barbro and Thylefors, Ingela (1996) *Om konflikter, hemma och på jobbet* (*On Conflicts at Home and at Work*). Stockholm: Natur och Kultur.

Lister, Ruth (2003) *Citizenship: Feminist Perspectives*, 2nd edn. Basingstoke and New York: Palgrave Macmillan.

Magnusson, Eva (1998) *Vardagens Könsinnebörder Under Förhandling: Om arbete, familj och produktion av kvinnlighet* (*Everyday Connotations of Gender in Negotiation: On Work, Family and Production of Femininity*). Umeå: Umeå Universitet.

Martinsson, Lena (1997) *Gemensamma liv: Om kön, kärlek och längtan* (*Shared Lives: On Gender, Love and Desire*). Stockholm: Carlssons Bokförlag.

Mauss, M. (1972 [1925]) *Gåvan* (*The Gift*). Uppsala: Argos.

Ministry of Health and Social Affairs Ds 2001: 57 (2001) *Barnafödandet i fokus: från befolkningspolitik till ett barnvänligt samhälle* (*Focus on childbirth: From Population Policy to a Child-friendly Society*). Stockholm: Fritzes.

Moxnes, Kari (1990) *Kjernesprengning i familien? Familieforandring ved samlivsbrudd og dannelse av nye samliv* (*Splitting the Nucleus of the Family? Family Change in Separation and Creation of New Ways of Living Together*). Oslo: Universitetsforlaget.

Nyman, Charlotte (2002) *Mine, Yours or Ours? Sharing in Swedish Couples*. Umeå: Umeå Universitet.

Okin, Susan (1989) *Justice, Gender, and the Family*. New York: Basic Books.

Pahl, Jan (1989) *Money and Marriage*. London: Macmillan.

Petrén, Gustaf and Ragnemalm, Hans (1980): *Sveriges grundlagar och tillhörande författningar med förklaringar. (The Instrument of Government in Sweden, with Statutes and Explanations)*, Stockholm: Liber förlag.

Plantin, Lars (2001) *Mäns föräldraskap: Om mäns upplevelser och erfarenheter av faderskapet* (*The Parenthood of Men: On Men's Experiences of Fatherhood*). Göteborg: Department of Social Work, Göteborg University.

Rapoport, Rhona and Rapoport, Robert (1976) *Dual-Career Families Re-examined: New Integrations of Work and Family*. London: Martin Robertson.

Regan, Milton C. (1999) *Alone Together: Law and Meanings of Marriage*. New York: Oxford University Press.

Risman, B. J. and Johnson-Sumerford, D. (1998) 'Doing it fairly: a study of postgender marriages', *Journal of Marriage and the Family* 60: 23–40.

Roman, Christine (1999) 'Familjelivets organisering – ekonomiska resurser, kön och manlig dominans' ('The organisation of family life – economic resources, gender and male dominance'), *Kvinnovetenskaplig tidskrift* 1: 3–20.

Roman, Christine and Vogler, Carolyne (1999) 'Managing money in British and Swedish Households', in *European Societies* 1(3): 419–456.

Schwartz, P. (1994) *Peer Marriage: How Love between Equals Really Works*. New York: Free Press.

Sevenhuijsen, Selma (1998) *Citizenship and the Ethics of Care: Feminist Considerations on Justice, Morality and Politics*. London: Routledge.

Simmel, Georg (1996 [1908]) 'Faithfulness and gratitude', in *The Gift: An Interdisciplinary Perspective*, (ed.) Aafte E. Komter. Amsterdam: Amsterdam University Press.

Skilsmässor och separationer – bakgrund och utveckling (Divorces and Separations – Background and Development). Demografiska rapporter 1995: 1 (Demographic reports 1995: 1). Stockholm: Statistiska Centralbyrån (Statistics Sweden).

Sprey, Jetsie (1979) 'Conflict theory and the study of marriage and the family', in *Contemporary Theory about the Family*, (eds) W. R. Burr, R. Hill, F. I. Nye, and I. Reiss. New York: Free Press.

Statistics Sweden (2003) Demografiska rapporter 2003 (Demographic Reports 2003). *Barn och deras familjer 2001 (Children and their Families 2001)*. Stockholm: Statistics Sweden.

Statistics Sweden, Demographic Reports 1995:1 (1995): *Skilsmässor och separationer – bakgrund och utveckling. (Divorces and Separations – Background and Developments.)* Örebro: Statistics Sweden

Sundström, Eva (2003) *Gender Regimes, Family Policies and Attitudes to Female Employment*. Doctoral thesis at the Department of Sociology, Umeå University.

Swedish Code of Statutes (Svensk författningssamling) 1996 (1997). Stockholm: Fritzes AB

Swedish Government Official Reports Series 1998:6 (1998): *Ty Makten Är Din (Because the Power is Yours)*. Stockholm: Fritzes.

Swedish Government Official Reports Series 2000:3 (2000): *Välfärd vid vägskäl. Utvecklingen under 1900-talet. (Welfare at Crossroads. The Development during the 1990s.)* Stockholm: Fritzes.

Swedish Government Official Reports Series 2001:79 (2001): *Välfärdsbokslut för 1990-talet. Kommittén Välfärdsbokslut. (Welfare Accounts for the 1990s. The Committee for Welfare Accounts.)* Stockholm: Fritzes.

Swedish Government Official Reports Series 2001:24 (2001): *Ur fattigdomsfällan. Slutbetänkande av Familjeutredningen. (Out of the Poverty Trap. Final Committee Report of the Family Inquiry.)* Stockholm: Fritzes.

Takahashi, Mieko (2003) *Gender Dimensions in Family Life: A Comparative Study of Structural Constraints and Power in Sweden and Japan*. Stockholm: Almquist and Wiksell International.

Thagaard, Tove (1996) *Arbeid, makt og kjælighet (Work, Power and Love)*. Bergen-Sandiken: Fagbokforlaget.

Théry, Irène (1993) *Le Démarriage (The End of Marriage)*. Paris: Odile Jacob.

Thylefors, Ingela (1996) 'Samspel, motspel, medspel – och Solospel' ('Playing with, for and against – and playing solo'), in *Om Konflikter hemma och på Jobbet (On Conflicts at Home and at Work)*, (eds) Barbro Lennéer-Axelsson and Ingela Thylefors. Stockholm: Natur och Kultur.

Wadsby, Marie and Swedin, Carl-Göran (1993) 'Skilsmässa – bakgrund och följder' ('Divorce – background and consequences'), in *Om modernt familjeliv och familjeseparationer: En antologi från ett forskarseminarium (On Modern Family Life and Family Separations: An Anthology from a Research Seminar)*, (eds) Anders Agell and Ulla Björnberg. Stockholm: Socialvetenskapliga forskningsrådet (Swedish Council for Working Life and Social Research).

Välfärd Vid Vägskäl. Delbetänkande/Kommittén Väfärdsbokslut. SOU 2000: 3 (Swedish Government Official Reports Series). Stockholm: Fritzes.

Välfärdsbokslut för 1990-talet. Kommittén Välfärdsbokslut. SOU 2001: 79 (Swedish Government Official Reports Series). Stockholm: Fritzes.

Waerness, Kari (1987) 'On the rationality of caring', in *Women and the State*, (ed.) Anne Showstack Sassoon. London: Hutchinson.

Van Yperen, Nico V. and Buunk, Bram P. (1994) 'Social comparison and social exchange in marital relationships', in *Entitlement and the Affectional Bond: Justice in Close Relationships*, (eds.) Melvin J. Lerner and Gerold Mikula. New York: Plenum Press.

Young, Michael and Willmott, Peter (1973) *The Symmetrical Family: A Study of Work and Leisure in the London Region*. Harmondsworth: Penguin.

Index

For Product Safety Concerns and Information please contact our EU
representative GPSR@taylorandfrancis.com
Taylor & Francis Verlag GmbH, Kaufingerstraße 24, 80331 München, Germany

www.ingramcontent.com/pod-product-compliance
Lightning Source LLC
Chambersburg PA
CBHW070244290326
41929CB00046B/2441